I0142758

Empowered Parenting:

Simple Strategies for Keeping Kids Healthy & Safe in a Complex World

A Nourished Minds' Publication

NOURISHED Minds
You Empowered...Life Improved

Copyright © 2016 by Nikole Seals

All rights reserved. No part of this publication may be reproduced, stored in a retrieval system, or transmitted in any form or by any means including electronic, mechanical, photocopying or recording, without the prior written permission of the publisher, nor be otherwise circulated in any form of binding or cover other than that in which it is published and without a similar condition being imposed on the subsequent purchaser. A limited quotation up to 500 words may be used for reference purposes with credits duly assigned.

First Printing: 2016

ISBN 978-0-9915063-2-3

This book was written for educational and informational purposes only. Suggestions and recommendations in this book are not intended to diagnose, prescribe, treat, or cure any disease, medical condition, or mental health condition and are not to be used as a substitute for regular health care. Any and all recommendations and advisements made by the author are not intended as treatment or prescription for any disease, medical condition, or mental health condition and use or application of said advisement and information is done so at the reader's own risk. Readers with symptoms of a medical condition or mental health condition should consult with a qualified physician or mental health practitioner. All readers of this book accept personal responsibility for the use of any information or advice. Any internet addresses printed in this book are provided as resources for which the author does not assume any responsibility for resource content. Readers assume any and all risk when visiting internet addresses printed in this book.

Published and distributed in the United States by Nourished Minds

www.NourishedMinds.com

Edited by Sally Casey

Author's Note

The names and identifying characteristics of people and places have been changed to protect and preserve the confidentiality of the people I have encountered as clients, their families, and the professionals with whom I have worked. Accounts are based on my recollections and experiences of certain events and may differ from the memories and perspectives of those involved in the actual events.

Dedication:

This book is dedicated to those family members and friends who always believed in me, even when I doubted myself. They supported my dreams and held me accountable. Without them, this book would have never made it to print. To my social worker friends who were in the trenches with me: thank you for the shoulders to cry on and the laughter to survive on.

I especially want to thank my clients and all of the families that allowed me into their lives and became the inspiration for this book. You were my best teachers.

Table of Contents

INTRODUCTION 1

1. WHO DOES SHE THINK SHE IS? 9

2. THE TOUGHEST JOB YOU CAN'T QUIT 17

3. THE COST OF CONVENIENCE 29

    How Empowered Parents Choose Foods: 39

4. THERE'S A PILL FOR THAT 51

    How Empowered Parents Manage Mental Health 65

5. THE GREAT DEBATE: VACCINES 75

    Being Empowered When It Comes to Vaccines 89

6. IN SICKNESS AND IN WEALTH 95

    How Empowered Parents Manage Healthcare 103

7. UPGRADING YOUR PARENTING SOFTWARE 113

    How Empowered Parents Manage Technology 119

8. THE NEW STRANGER DANGER 129

    How Empowered Parents Protect Their Kids 139

9. IT TAKES A VILLAGE...AND AN OCCASIONAL GLASS OF WINE 149

RESOURCE LIST 153

BIBLIOGRAPHY 163

INTRODUCTION

Theresa is a single mom of an eight-year old boy. Like most single mothers, she tries to manage the delicate balancing act of being a primary caregiver, full-time employee, friend, and daughter to aging parents. As if that wasn't enough, she has also experienced the daily heartbreak of watching her son suffer. He had a painful, unsightly, unexplained rash on his hands and feet. To add insult to injury, her son was teased relentlessly by his classmates. The rash would often get inflamed and spread from his fingertips down to the back of his hands. Covering his hands was not an option since gloves seemed to make matters worse. As a resident of sunny southern California, Theresa knew that sending him to school in a pair of mittens would officially declare her child a freak show.

Theresa came to me for advice after several frustrating visits to her family pediatrician. Her own doctor, who had known her son since birth, basically shrugged his shoulders and dismissed her with a prescription for cortisone cream. She spent a few late nights searching the internet for answers but found that the massive amounts of contradictory information only added to her frustrations. She was desperate for a solution.

As a health educator, I'm fairly knowledgeable when it comes to nutrition, physiology and how the body works. But I am not a doctor, nor do I attempt to make any diagnosis of disease or prescribe treatments. What I do is to help parents find answers and solutions by exploring their options and getting proactive. Just because Theresa's pediatrician didn't have an answer didn't mean there wasn't an answer. What I explained to Theresa was that rashes are the body's way of telling us that something is not right. Typically, we get sick or present with symptoms because either one of two things are happening: 1) The body is reacting to an exposure like a virus or an external trigger that we have taken in by skin or mouth like a chemical or allergen, or 2) The body is responding to a deficiency like a lack of water, oxygen, or nutrients. Instead of just focusing on eliminating the symptom like most physicians are trained to do, we set out to discover the "origin" of her son's problem.

For that I referred her to a naturopathic physician, which was something new for her. Naturopaths base their practice of healthcare on the belief that the body has a natural ability to heal itself when given what it needs. Together as a team, we were able to figure out that her son has some deficiencies that had made him susceptible to a viral infection. She opted to use natural remedies to treat the infection while making changes to his diet in order to boost his clearly suppressed immune system. She managed to greatly reduce her son's flare ups to once or twice a year and now she's able to stop the rashes from spreading altogether. But the most awesome part of the story is that Theresa is now empowered to handle whatever parenting challenges come her way. Her experience boosted her confidence and made her feel totally capable of managing her child's health. Better yet, she no longer feels intimidated by her pediatrician and knows that she has options. She's the perfect example of what being an *Empowered Parent* is all about.

If you are reading this, you're keenly aware of how insanely challenging it is to be a parent in today's world. Aside from your basic duties of keeping your child alive and healthy, you're now required to be a doctor, scientist, and tech support. Plus, you get to waste endless hours of your time sifting through conflicting information online, only to discover that you're more confused than ever. Is gluten really bad? Should I keep giving my child antibiotics? Is my teen sexting? Will I ever get eight hours of sleep again?

You can torture yourself with these types of questions and feed into that growing sense of self-doubt and fear, or you can decide that it's an exhausting way to live and you want better for yourself and your family. The truth is—it doesn't have to be complicated. We allow confusion, misinformation, and dependence on external "experts" to throw us off course. We are constantly underestimating our own abilities to make good choices and to raise healthy kids. The question you really need to be asking yourself is, "Am I ready to start trusting my own abilities and take back my power and control? I hope you answered yes because that's exactly what this book will help you to do.

Raising Kids on Fast Forward

Is time flying by or am I the only one who feels like life is on warp speed? In a rare moment of downtime, I happened to catch the 1998 Will Smith movie, *Enemy of the State*, on some random digital channel (I'm one of those diehards who refuse to pay for cable so I pick up free digital channels with TV antennas. Remember when TV was free?). When the movie first came out, it seemed so ridiculous to think that there were cameras everywhere that could capture our every move. After all, we live in the US and we would never allow for that type of egregious violation of our privacy. Fast forward fifteen years and there are now cameras everywhere. Satellite cameras can zoom in on real-time pictures of our homes. Google knows that I got lost in the "bad" part of town while trying to find a short-cut to the airport last month. Target not only tracks what we buy and how we pay for it but then records it all on video for quality assurance purposes.

> Today's kids face challenges unlike any other generation in our history.

The point is that we've come a long way in a relatively short period of time. In fact, we have experienced more growth and change in the past thirty years than we have in the history of the world. We owe that in a large part to the rapid advancement in technology that makes us feel as if our world changed overnight. One day we're tethered to a phone in the wall and the next, we're walking down the street video chatting with a friend in Dubai on a mini hand-held computer.

While advancements in industry, technology and medicine have improved our lives, they have also complicated the job of raising healthy kids and keeping them safe. Even if you are lucky enough to have great parents, and managed to absorb all of their wisdom, it will only get you so far. Think about the advice you get from your own parents; practical and maybe even useful at times, but what does your mom know about sexting, cyber bullying, or Pharm parties?

Today's kids face challenges unlike any other generation in our history. This means that as a parent, you are expected to know how to handle these new challenges and manage 21st century problems. Think of your knowledge and skills as the software you use to make decisions and take action. Is your software up-to-date? Many parents are running on outdated software and forget that they need to constantly upgrade to the latest version in order to stay informed. Failure to do so results in frustration, self-doubt, and a sense that you are no longer in control.

Over the years, I've heard a common complaint from parents who feel as if they are losing control of their kids. And I don't just mean not being able to manage a child's behavior. I'm talking about companies deciding what your child eats, doctors labeling and medicating your child, and government mandates telling you what you can and can't do with your own family. When you depend on these external forces to guide your decisions, you set yourself up to be misled or manipulated. This dependent type of thinking will eventually strip you of all your power and leave you feeling helpless.

The Fear Factor

The most important insight I gained during my career as a social worker was in understanding the profound impact that fear has on a parent's choices and decisions. Many parents live in fear: fear that their child will get a life threatening illness or injury; will do poorly in school; won't make friends; will get addicted to drugs; will be sexually active too early; or will be abducted or a victim of violence. That's just the short list and unfortunately, all of these are valid concerns and reflective of the time we live in.

Such fears can be overwhelming and paralyzing even for the most skilled and experienced parent. I have counseled many parents who suffer from anxiety, depression, and sleeplessness because they are in constant state of worry over all the "what ifs?" and uncertainty. When you add to this all the normal stressors of being an adult and having to support a family, the result is one very anxious and exhausted human being.

The problem is that when you're frustrated, overwhelmed, and anxious; you become an easy for manipulation by all the external influences that bombard us each day. *Most of the time, we are totally unaware of these influences.* Let me give you an example. Have you noticed the major increase in prescription drug commercials in recent years? It's hard not to! They pop up everywhere: TV, Youtube videos, magazines, and even while listening to your favorite music app. Say you briefly see an ad (5 to 10 seconds is all it takes) for depression and think to yourself, "How annoying". You don't pay it much attention. Or so you think.

One year later you discover your teenage daughter is bullied at school and tells you she sometimes feels like she wants to die. She seems sad and depressed, so you immediately take her in for counseling. The therapist recommends putting your daughter on an ant-depressant. At that very moment, that advertisement for an anti-depressant will pop into your head. Next thing you know, the therapist is not only giving your daughter a prescription but she gladly gives you one too…you know, to help "get through" this rough time.

I'm not saying it's wrong to decide to manage that situation with prescription drugs. What I am suggesting is that you owe it to yourself and your child to explore your options, get the facts, and make informed decisions.

I didn't write this book to tell you how to raise your kids. Having worked as a social worker and family counselor, I already know that you are the "expert." No one else knows your children better than you. So if you're looking for someone to tell you how to parent, I'm not the one. What I can help with is to show you how to manage your job as a parent in a way that will reduce your fears and increase your confidence. I can help you to be an informed consumer and teach you effective strategies to manage the challenges of living in a high-tech, profit-driven, environmentally toxic, violence-prone, medication nation.

> ➤ It's about no longer allowing your fears and uncertainties to influence your decisions.
>
> ➤ It's about being proactive instead of reactive.
>
> ➤ It's about being informed rather than being influenced.
>
> ➤ It's about being an *Empowered Parent*.

How This Book Will Help You

You can apply the information in this book to parenting children of all ages. I will give specific information and facts as they relate to different age groups. For example, when we discuss nutrition, we'll talk about the specific needs of young children, preteens, and teenagers. You can read straight through or skip the information you don't think is applicable to your child's age.

You may pick up on the fact that I'm fairly blunt. I think sugar-coating things makes an assumption that you're not strong enough to hear the truth. I know we've never met, but if you chose to read this book then I must believe you're the type of person who likes a straight shooter. Don't be thrown off by my candor or my tendency to emphasize my point with some mild profanity.

I'm also a true believer in the power of laughter and often use humor as a way to neutralize fear and anxiety. I have been using humor as a counselor and in my workshops for many years and have found it to be far more effective than any pill.

Of course the optimal time to read this book is before you have children. This way, you know what you're getting yourself into, plus, you're more likely to have a quiet, private space to relax. If you're already a parent, then you lost your privacy a long time ago and will have to find a place to hide and read this book in snippets. Maybe you'll find time in your car during lunch or after you've read *Goodnight Moon* to your child for the 100th time.

I believe in the old African proverb that it takes a village to raise a child. Parenting should be a collective effort because it is such a demanding job. You may not recognize it but family members, friends, teachers, and even people on social media can influence your parenting. I wrote this book for parents (grandparents, foster parents, guardians) and for all those who play a supporting role (friends, educators, social workers, counselors). We all need to upgrade our software. Your success is largely dependent on the people with whom you surround yourself. I like to call them your "supporting cast." If their information is faulty or outdated, then they will bring more confusion and frustration into your life. The information in this book is for the benefit of both those who are raising kids *and* their support systems such as teachers and counselors. The type of changes needed to make this world a safer, healthier place for our kids require a group effort.

An empowered individual can change their life but an empowered community of individuals can change the world.

Let me give you a preview of how this book will help you on the individual level. In following chapters:

- You'll learn the truth about the food your children eat, the medicines prescribed to them, and how these things affect their health, physical development, and emotional well-being.

- You'll discover the ways that the food and drug industries have fooled you into buying their products, despite knowing that their products are hazardous to your child's health and development. You'll learn which companies and brands to avoid and which companies you can trust.

- We'll discuss how our own government is failing to protect our kids and how your rights as a parent are slowly being eroded and ignored.

- We'll take an in-depth look at how our healthcare system is one of the biggest threats to your child's safety and wellness and what you can do to protect your family.

- We'll examine the pros and cons of technology and discuss how it impacts your child's development, safety, and self-identity. You'll learn how to effectively manage and supervise your child's use of technology.

- You'll get the tools you need to create a prevention and safety plan so that you can prevent or manage a problem or crisis.

By the time you finish this book, you'll be informed and fully equipped with the tools and resources you need to protect, nourish and care for your family. This book will empower you to make confident decisions and help you to raise healthy, happy children. Soon, you'll experience the power of knowledge and the confidence that comes from knowing that you have it all under control. I can't promise you a life free from stress, but you will make smarter decisions, worry less, eat better, save money, and trust yourself more. That's the *Empowered Parenting* way.

Before we get started I need to remind you of one thing. It takes a smart and courageous parent to acknowledge the need for support and to invest rare "free" moments into reading a book. I thank you for spending your time with me. You are my inspiration for writing this book.

CH. 1 – WHO DOES SHE THINK SHE IS?

My very first job at the wise old age of sixteen was as a youth counselor with the YMCA. I loved everything about it. In my mind I was getting paid to play. I always had a natural ability and an innate desire to work with kids, even when I was still a kid myself. Over the years I rose up the ranks and eventually became a site director. It meant less time on the playground and more time doing program development and interacting with parents. When parents were late picking up their kids or got behind on their payments, I would have to pull them aside and enforce the rules.

To my surprise, parents started opening up to me and telling me about their problems. I was only twenty years old at the time. Yet, here were these much older adults coming to me with their real-life problems, asking for my advice. The crazy thing is that I was totally comfortable with it and was in my element. Sure, I had no point of reference except my own childhood experiences, but there I was talking marital problems, unemployment, and depression with anyone who needed a sympathetic ear. I didn't know it then, but I was social worker before I even knew what it meant to be a social worker.

The road to officially becoming a social worker was a natural progression. By age twenty-four, I had my degree in human services and child development and went to work for a county agency as a counselor for abused children. That job was like being in boot camp before heading off to war. I was responsible for the supervision and care of children who had become wards of the juvenile court system. However, my more important role was to help them cope with the abuse they had suffered and the resulting separation from their families. It was intense and emotionally demanding. I felt like I lived with these children; going home only to sleep, change clothes, and return for another day. The kids often looked to us as parents since some of them stayed with us for years or would return back to us after a failed placement with foster parents. Sometimes they would get attached to us and not want to go back home. Other times they came to us angry, distrustful, broken, and scared.

The county agency was where I learned about the long-term effects that trauma has on a child. It's difficult for children to process pain and trauma. They either lack the verbal skills to communicate what they are feeling or the mental comprehension to understand it. Even teens struggle with it because they experience such a heightened state of emotions and tend to internalize. Those that internalized their pain came to us depressed or anxious, or in severe cases, would inflict harm to themselves. Then you had the kids who expressed their pain physically. They would hit, kick, throw stuff, spit, or destroy things around the house. I had to break up fights, talk teenagers off the roof, stay up all night to monitor children on suicide watch, and talk kids out of running away. I was spit on twice, had my hair pulled out once, got the chicken pox, and became an expert at nit combing after several outbreaks of head lice.

I'd like to note that none of this was in the job description. My employer was wise to omit the "unforeseen" physical demands of the job because no one in their right mind would knowingly sign up for this shit. My friends and family thought I was crazy for staying. They couldn't understand what I liked about it. "It's so depressing," they would say. Truth is, I didn't like it. I loved it. It was hard, consuming, physically and emotionally taxing work, but it had its rewards.

I felt compelled to show these children what a trustworthy, loving caretaker should look and act like. They had lost faith and trust in adults and I wanted to restore their faith. I wanted them to have an example of a positive role model in their lives. So many kids grow up thinking that hitting, yelling, fighting, and using drugs is normal parental behavior. I wanted them to know otherwise. I wanted them to know they could grow up to act and be something different.

For two years, I worked in the nursery with infants and toddlers. It was not uncommon for newborn babies to come directly from the hospital because their mother used drugs during her pregnancy. These precious, fragile little souls experienced more trauma in their short three days of life than some of us do in a lifetime. Can you imagine being a baby and being addicted to heroin?! For those of you who don't know, babies who are addicted to drugs go through

[10]

the same type of withdrawal symptoms as adults. They get sick, vomit, shake, tremor, and struggle to fall sleep.

By far one of the most difficult things I have ever done in my life is to hold a drug-addicted newborn in my arms for hours on end while they shrieked and suffered through violent tremors. At times, when it was dark and my co-workers couldn't see me, I cried too. My heart ached for those babies, but I know I needed to move past my own emotions and be there for them. I was so determined to remain patient and gentle despite my urges to bang my head against the wall.

That type of crying for such long periods of time can make you snap…if you let it. I remember I use to whisper into the babies' ears with a sweet, soft, angelic voice and say stuff like, "You're killing me," or "Why do you hate me so much?" It made me laugh, it made my co-workers laugh, and like a soothing lullaby, our laughter calmed the babies. My practice of laughter therapy was born in that nursery and would become my most powerful tool for facing the challenges that lie ahead.

I'd be lying if I said I never let myself get attached. I did all the time, but over the years I learned how to put up my guard and keep my emotions in check. It was necessary as a way to protect myself and to help the kids cope with reality that our relationship would eventually come to an end. Healthy termination, we called it.

I wanted to save each and every one of those kids. I had this strong desire and need to protect them. I started talking to their social workers to learn more about their cases and figure out ways to help them. It was during one of these conversations that a coworker suggested I consider getting my master's degree in social work. It wasn't the first time the thought crossed my mind, but it had always dissipated when I thought about the cost of going back to school. She explained that agency I worked for would assist with the cost as long as I returned to work post-graduation. *"I get my degree and I'll have a job to come back to too?"* I asked in disbelief. Six months later, I was accepted to the School of Social Work Program at my local university.

Graduate school was a blur. I was in a constant state of absorbing information and regurgitating it in a way that made sense. I learned an enormous amount of book knowledge regarding theory, policy, treatment modalities, cultural diversity, and program development. Unfortunately, very little of it would prepare me for the next ten years of my life. I don't want to minimize the value of my education, but nothing comes close to the lessons you get from hands- on experience.

During my second year of graduate school, I was offered the rare opportunity of being an intern in the Child Welfare Department—more specifically Child Protective Services. It was rare because they typically didn't allow students to perform this job. Knowing what I know now, I couldn't agree more. It's like a cadet showing up to the police academy, giving him a gun and a badge, and wishing him "good luck out there." What surprised everyone, including me, was that my previous experience of getting abused by abused kids had made me quite fearless and tolerant.

Two months after graduation, I was offered a bona fide full-time position with the Child Welfare Department. After one year of being a rookie, I accepted a position with a local law enforcement agency to be their resident social worker. I would become a part of their detective bureau that investigated crimes against children. And yes…it was exactly as it sounds—like working on an episode of COPS.

The practice of social workers and law enforcement partnering up was a new concept, so the boundaries weren't cemented. I became very close with the detectives that I worked with. They came to depend on me, which made me feel valued. What you may not know about law enforcement is that they really don't like dealing with cases that involve child abuse, mental illness, or domestic violence. They are trained to keep the peace, assess if a crime has occurred, and gather evidence. Dealing with the emotional aspects of cases is not their forte.

Crisis intervention was my specialty and word quickly spread from the detectives to patrol that I was good with diffusing emotionally-charged family situations. What started out as just case consultations soon graduated to ride-alongs and early morning call-outs. I thought nothing of driving out to drug motels at two in the morning to meet officers. Part of the reason was that once I learned the details of situation, it was useless to try and go back to bed. It's hard to fall asleep when you know there's a three-year-old child found abandoned in a dirty motel room. I also did it because I trusted those officers with my life and knew they would protect me.

I really felt like I was making a difference. All the drama and stress seemed worth it when I thought I was helping a child to live a life free from abuse. Then the true reality of my work set in and it changed everything.

Friend or Foe

At the request of an officer, I visited a home to investigate an allegation of physical abuse. Physical abuse cases are not as common as most people think. Of all reported cases of maltreatment in the U.S., only about 18 percent are reports of physical abuse (US Dept. Health and Human Services, 2013). They are easier to prove/disprove since injuries make for strong evidence, but depending on the severity of the injury, they can also be very emotionally-charged investigations.

[12]

I remember that the officer seemed very relieved to see me when I pulled up to the home. He had explained that there were approximately fifteen relatives inside with one female victim who I'll refer to as Annie. I met privately with Annie and did my best to make her feel safe and comfortable. She was five and adorable. Her hair was parted down the middle and fingered-combed into two pigtails; making the walnut-sized patches of missing hair easy to see. She had this sweet carved pumpkin grin that made her lisp when she answered my questions. Not even all of that cuteness could detract from the enormous purple bruise on the left side of her petite face. It looked exactly like a drawing of thanksgiving turkey you'd trace from your hand; except it was an adult sized handprint. I remember taking notice of how the fingertips of the bruise extended into her hairline.

Her family members were rightfully upset after having discovered Annie's injuries. The scene inside the house was chaotic and hostile with many of the male relatives wanting to seek their own form of vigilante justice. I had managed to calm the group long enough for them to explain that Annie's mother had shown up at the house that day after being "missing in action" for the past two weeks. They told me they confronted the mom about Annie's injuries and she left the home in a panic. Family members had gathered together to discuss how to handle the situation and decided it was best to call the police.

After interviewing Annie and her family, it was clear that mom's boyfriend was responsible for the abuse. Mom had only recently started dating this man and the family hated him. He had turned the mother on to drugs and didn't like Annie because she was another man's child. The officer immediately jumped into action to locate the mom and her boyfriend and bring them in for questioning. I on the other hand began the process of determining where Annie would be safe.

Here's where it gets complicated. State mandates required us to try to place children with relatives when temporarily removed from a parent's care. In the case of Annie, I had five adult relatives in that house who were willing to be her caretaker. Unfortunately, the state mandate also holds these relative caretakers to a ridiculously high standard. Based on state law, the relatives would need to provide Annie with her own room, her own bed, and pass a home safety inspection and criminal background check. The state made us use the same requirements needed to approve foster homes for relative's homes. It was unrealistic and unfair.

To this day, it is so painful to think about what I ended up doing to Annie and her family. Of the five relatives, only one passed the background check. They each had some type of criminal charge in their history that, according to state mandates, ruled them out as possible caretakers. The remaining relative

[13]

lived in a one-bedroom apartment shared by four people, which was unacceptable to the state of California.

I was informed by my supervisor that I could not leave Annie with any of her relatives. I had to break the news to those family members, and even worse, tell them that I would be taking Annie with me and placing her in a foster home. They had put their trust in me to help and then I broke that trust and they hated me for it. I hated me too, and I knew it wasn't right. They loved that little girl, and I had no doubt that every single one of them would have protected her with their lives. And Annie…she was safe with them. She wasn't afraid of them. Because of a technicality with the law, I had to take her from them. I was a stranger to her, and I took her from the people she knew and trusted and placed her with more strangers. I took her from her old nightmare and put her in a new one.

In that moment, I felt like I had become a part of the nightmare that I was trying to protect kids from. It nearly destroyed me. I became increasingly resentful of my employers and the flawed system that seemed designed to punish the victims. I felt powerless. My co-workers and friends kept telling me that I was just doing my job—that I didn't have a choice. That only seemed to make me angrier. I became cynical, hardened, and detached. It was the only way I was able to wake up each morning and do my job. Quitting wasn't an option because each day, new cases landed on my desk which meant there were still kids and families that I *might* be able to help.

I'm aware that this is why some people hate child protective social workers and the reason why social workers seemed detached and uncaring. You start off wanting to save the world and eventually end up with your hands tied by the bureaucratic red tape of our broken child welfare system. Management, so far removed from the reality of the people's lives, were the ones making the final decisions. They wanted workers to do as told, even if it went against a worker's values and better judgment. The workers who got with the program got promoted. Others chose not to ruffle any feathers and just did their jobs. I realized I had other options.

When you know you have choices and believe in your ability to make good decisions, that kind of freedom and internal trust makes you feel powerful. That is how empowerment works.

[14]

Having options and choices puts you back in the driver's seat of your own life. When we let others dictate what we do and how we think, we become dependent on them; whether it's the government, our employer, or our family doctor. I couldn't give in to that type of dependency and victim mentality. I needed to be able to live with myself. I needed to stay true to my commitment to not only protect kids, but to protect and serve their families as well. I decided that I didn't want to work for the government; I wanted to work for families. I figured that my best chance of staying in control was to become very knowledgeable and really good at what I did.

I became well versed on the laws, mandates, and protocols so that I knew how to use them or work my way around them. I shared this information with families so that they could better navigate the system. I tried to know more than management because it's hard to argue about things you don't understand. I learned that management would sooner agree with me than acknowledge that they didn't understand something. I would find all kinds of creative ways to keep kids in their homes. I'd help parent's child-proof their homes or have kids go into respite care with friends while parents made their homes inhabitable again. I conducted trainings for mandated reporters to try to reduce the number of unjustified reports filed against parents. I even started giving child abuse trainings at high schools so teens knew the difference between abuse and disciplinary action. I fought hard for the things I believed in. The more informed I was, the more independence I got.

I didn't win every battle, and in the later part of my seventeen-year career with the agency, I had some horrific experiences that made it no longer worth the fight. In 2010, I chose to resign. The thought of walking away from my friends, good benefits, and what I thought was job security scared the Hell out of me, but sometimes we have to walk into our fears.

In my quest to have different experiences, I spent three years working as a clinical social worker doing individual and group therapy for families in crisis and recovery. I spent another three years enhancing my knowledge and finding ways to improve family services by working as a program manager for two well-known non-profits in Los Angeles County. I also pursued and accomplished my dream of being a writer and researcher when I joined EBSCO Publishing, one of the largest online educational publishing companies. If I hadn't listened to my discontent, I would have missed out on amazing opportunities to learn and become better at what I do. Twenty-five years of hard work and the life-changing experiences that were associated with it provided me with the growth that I needed to launch my own coaching practice and online publishing company, Nourished Minds.

The most valuable information I learned was from parents and co-workers. I was fortunate to work with some of the most amazing, caring professionals who are still my friends to this day. Child Protective Services (CPS) social workers are some of the most hated people in this country; second only to the IRS. I blame the media. In every news story, TV show, or movie, the social worker is the villain; an unattractive, coldhearted, cynical woman who acts as judge and jury. She's always holding files and dresses like a librarian.

Think I'm exaggerating? Did you see the movie *Losing Isaiah* with Halle Berry? The social worker in that movie was mean and dowdy and had files with her at all times. In the award-winning movie, *Precious,* Mariah Carey played the role of the social worker. They actually used make-up to make her appear unattractive. And true to form, her character was also dowdy, mean, and had a desk stacked with files. Hopefully you're starting to realize that this is not reality.

What you read in the newspaper should also be questioned. I worked on many high profile cases involving serious crimes against children. Reporters would call and try to trick me into divulging information about the investigation. "No comment," I'd say. Next day I'd read about the case in the newspaper and half of the story would be complete lies. Since they were never able to get information out of workers (we were bound by rules of conduct), they would just make stuff up. I think part of the problem is that there has always been so much secrecy about this type of social work and about child abuse investigations. The secrecy has led to misconceptions about social workers having power to break up families for no reason.

I could write an entire book on my work experiences but don't want to take up any more of our time together. We've got a lot to cover. My point in sharing my story with you is that you should always qualify the people you take advice from. When it comes down to it, the credentials and letters behind someone's name often don't matter.

I've worked with psychiatrists who abuse medications, doctors that are obese, dentists with bad teeth, and police officers whose kids are in and out of juvenile hall. Degrees and licenses are not strong indicators of a professional's level of experience or expertise. You must get to know them. Find out what they've done and where they've been. Ask them questions. Get an understanding of their beliefs and values and then decide if they are in alignment with yours. Only then should you consider taking their advice.

My hope is that you feel I'm qualified to take you on this truth-discovering journey. Are you ready to embrace your personal power and be the one calling the shots when it comes to your own family?

CH. 2 – THE TOUGHEST JOB YOU CAN'T QUIT

Rose Kennedy said, "When you hold your baby in your arms for the first time, and you think of all the things you can say and do to influence him, it is a tremendous responsibility. What you do with him can not only influence him, but everyone he meets and not for a day or a month or a year, but for time and eternity." Whoa, Rose! That's what I call a verbal contraception. Talk about a reality check. They should engrave this quote on a plaque and hang it over the entry way to every high school and bar in the country. Parenting is by far the most important job a person will perform in their lifetime and Rose Kennedy was right; it shouldn't be taken lightly. I know some people don't like it when parenting is referred to as a job but I call it like I see it. It is a labor of love but it can also be a daily grind. Like most jobs, it requires a unique set of skills and a willingness to learn.

Think of it this way; as a parent you need to adjust and adapt your skills and practices to keep up with each new advancement, social issue, and threat to your child's safety. So basically every year you keep having more responsibilities added to your job description.

I'm unaware of any official human-resource-approved job description for being a parent, but let's pretend one exists. How might that *want ad* look today in comparison to an ad placed in the 1970s?

Seeking: Full-time caretaker for lifetime commitment
Job Title: Parent
Start date: August 8, 1972

Responsibilities: Provide child(ren) with basic needs of food, water, shelter; maintain adequate supervision; ensure child is properly educated; set rules and boundaries to help child become a law abiding citizen; role model gender-specific roles to help child develop healthy self-identity and learn how to engage with others
Skills: Applicant must possess the ability to prepare foods, maintain a home, enforce discipline, teach children morals and values, and provide emotional support

Baby Boomers may or may not agree that it was a simpler time back then. Raising children was a family affair. Most families were two-parent households and it was not unusual to have grandparents living in the home or somewhere close by. Although many women worked outside of the home, the dual role of *bringing home the bacon and frying it up in a pan* had not yet become the norm.

Fast food restaurants were becoming popular options to home cooked meals, yet some food companies still delivered fresh produce and dairy to people's homes. Schools were solely responsible for educating kids, so parents weren't required to spend three hours each night working on homework. There were only thirteen strictly-censored TV channels. Seatbelts and helmets were suggested but not required. There was less traffic which meant less time commuting, yet there seemed to be far more martini drinking.

Andrea O'Reilly, author and an associate professor in the women's studies department at Toronto's York University would agree. The 1970s was a pivotal era for women; the image of the "proper wife was collapsing" and children had yet to become "all-consuming 'projects', doomed for failure if they weren't read six stories at bedtime" (O'Reilly, 2013).

Now let's fast forward to today's job description.

Seeking: Full-time caretaker for lifetime commitment
Job Title: Parent
Start date: March 8, 2016

Responsibilities: Provide child(ren) with foods free of harmful chemicals and carcinogens and a water source that is free of chlorine, heavy metals, and traces of prescription medication; provide a clean, safe home free

[18]

from asbestos, lead, and toxins but with a strong Wi-Fi signal so children can stay connected to the world; maintain adequate supervision despite the fact that strangers can enter your home through phones and computers; ensure child is properly educated on new curriculum that you can't begin to understand; set rules and boundaries to help entitled children learn the value of money and to respect others despite the fact that your child is constantly exposed to media content and behaviors that promote materialism, vanity, and disrespect; role model gender-specific roles to help child develop healthy self-identity in a gender-neutral society; and learn how to research, diagnose and treat all minor medical conditions.

Skills: Must possess ability to manage full-time job and role as primary caretaker; act as cook, nutritionist, housekeeper, nurse, tutor, disciplinarian, taxi driver, soccer coach, advocate, school volunteer, family mediator, detective, drug and alcohol counselor, sex educator, internet security expert, LGBT expert, violence prevention task force, and the FCC (Federal Communication Commission)

Sound about right? We must admit that life has gotten easier in many ways. We are fortunate to live in a prosperous time where technology gives us limitless access to information and allows us to connect with others in ways we never imagined possible.

Medicine has extended our lives and food has never been more abundant. Modernization has afforded us many benefits and we pay dearly for them. This "fast-acting," "long-lasting," "great-tasting" world we live in has cost us the very thing we desire most: control. The control that we have willingly handed over to the food, drug, tech, and medical industries has enabled them to have a significant influence on our lives.

> **This "fast-acting," "long-lasting," "great-tasting" world we live in has cost us the very thing we desire most: control.**

These industries have managed to keep us entertained, drugged up, sick, or too confused to take notice of the fact that they have become more powerful than our own government. When you are responsible for raising another human life, you don't always have time to advocate for your family and play watchdog. Keeping you confused and scared is a great way to control you.

In his New York Times best-selling book, *Predictably Irrational (2008)*, MIT professor Dan Ariely surmises that "behavioral economists believe that people are susceptible to irrelevant influences from their immediate environment, irrelevant emotions, shortsightedness, and other forms of irrationality." Companies spend millions of dollars each year trying to better understand and predict our irrational behaviors. Yes, you have been the proverbial rat in a decades-long study designed to better understand your habits and buying behaviors so they can be exploited for a profit.

At the same time, companies within these different industries work very hard to make sure you stay loyal to their products and services. They use faulty science to convince you and fear to keep you from seeking the truth. They keep getting richer while families are just trying to keep their heads above water. As a matter of fact, big business is hoping that you are way too stressed out, tired, and confused to discover the truth. They'd much rather tell you what to think, but you will never be able to take ownership of your life if you keep your blinders on.

To get a better understanding of how each of these industries has grown to become such powerful influences in our daily lives, let's briefly examine each one individually.

The Food Industry

The food industry is comprised of the people and companies that grow our food and provide the farming materials (agriculture), the companies that process and ship our food (manufacturers and distributors), and the companies that sell food to us (marketers and retail).

We, the consumers, are the people who keep all these other people in business. We buy food because we need it to live and because we like to eat. We like food so much that on average, we each spend over $6,000 annually on food and make 1.6 trips to the grocery store every week: that's how the US food retail industry managed to bring in 5.27 trillion dollars in 2014 (Sloan, 2014).

If food is in such great abundance, why are Americans so unhealthy? If the food industry is experiencing trillions of dollars in sales, why are 15.8 million children living in a household with limited access to adequate food, and why do nearly half (49 percent) of American children consume diets that don't even meet the basic recommendations made by the 2010 USDA Dietary Guidelines?

We'll be answering these questions and more in the next chapter. We'll also explore the many ways that we as consumers are manipulated and lied to on a daily basis. You'll learn how to be a smarter consumer and build confidence in your ability to find healthy products amidst all the hype.

[20]

FUN FOOD STATS

- *American families seem to favor snacks above all else resulting in about 41.4 billion dollars of sales in 2010 (Statista, 2010).*

- *Our snack of choice...salty snacks. Our love for treats that raise our blood pressure experienced one of the highest growth in sales in 2013 (Statista, 2013).*

- *When it comes to fast food we still prefer McDonalds, then Subway. Not surprisingly Starbucks coming in at a close third (Technomic, 2013).*

- *Half of adults bought prepared foods at a convenience store in 2013. (Hanson, 2013) Seriously? My guess is that this same half of adults spent 25 percent of their post-lunch time in the bathroom.*

- *Eight in ten family dinners involve adults only and no kids under the age of eighteen (U.S. Census Bureau, 2010).*

- *Fifty-six percent of home cooks made at least one weeknight dinner from scratch, with poultry as the meat of choice and the most popular vegetables being tomatoes onions and potatoes. (Multisponsor Surveys, Inc, 2012).*

- *In 2012, vitamins became the number one nutritional specialty item being purchased with one in five moms making an effort to include probiotics (mostly in the form of yogurt) into their child's diet. (MSI, 2012).*

The Drug Industry

We love a quick fix. Americans take full advantage of modern day medicine to cure our physical and emotional ailments. While we love the fast-acting, mind-altering, problem-solving effects of drugs, we don't always appreciate the price we have to pay for these magic potions.

While the most common form of "drugs" are food, sugar, and caffeine; for the purpose of this discussion we are going to strictly focus on pharmaceutical drugs, both over-the-counter and prescription. Our dependence on these drugs is wreaking havoc on our minds, bodies, finances, and families. This is going to be your wakeup call.

Now before some of you go and get your panties in a bunch thinking that I'm criticizing the use of all medicines, let me be clear: I am truly grateful for emergency, lifesaving medicine. I rank it at the top of the list of humankind's greatest contributions. Medicine has saved people that I love, kept children from dying, and helped to increase the human lifespan. I don't hate all drugs.

What I'm fundamentally opposed to is the corporate agenda of keeping Americans drugged and dependent. I have nothing but contempt for the greed and utter lack of concern for human life that, like a tumor, has grown and taken over the drug industry. Don't just take my word for it, though. Let's look at the facts.

The business of making drugs and getting people dependent on drugs is highly profitable. Pharmaceutical companies are responsible for the development, production and marketing of drugs. Pfizer is the largest pharmaceutical company in the world. In 2012, Pfizer reported a total annual revenue of 60 billion dollars; 47 billion from pharmaceutical sales alone (Statista, 2012). Cancer drugs are the best-selling drugs, raking in 60 billion dollars worldwide in 2012 (Statista, 2012).

The Cost for Americans

Americans filled about 4.3 billion prescriptions in 2014 at the cost of about 374 billion dollars (Time, 2014). In 2011, Americans made an estimated 2,301,059 visits to hospital emergency rooms across the country for adverse reactions to pharmaceutical drugs (both prescribed and over-the-counter). Over 500,000 of these visits were due to reactions from antivirals and antibiotics like penicillin, while 362,000 visits were for reactions to pain relievers. (Substance Abuse Mental Health Services Administration, 2011).

Which Medicines Pose the Greatest Risks?	
Children Under Age 4	**Preteens & Teens**
Ibuprofen, acetaminophen, multi-vitamins, diaper rash products, anti-fungal creams, cold medicines, laxatives	Multi-vitamins, ibuprofen, acetaminophen, antihistamines, anti-anxiety meds, anti-psychotic meds

Kids are most likely to find these drugs in their own homes in these common places: on the ground or misplaced; in a purse or wallet; on top of a counter, dresser or nightstand; in an unsecure medicine cabinet; or in a pill box or bag of pills.

Approximately 1.34 million calls are made to poison control centers for children each year; 81% of calls are for children who accidentally ingested a drug while 19% are for children that were over medicated or given the wrong medicine (SafeKids.org)

One in four teens think it's okay to use prescription drugs as a study aid; need to study is the primary motive for misuse, despite data that links such drug use to low grade point averages (Drug Free, 2012).

The ultimate goal of this book is to increase your awareness and proactivity. Medicines are a necessity of life, but we don't always choose and use them responsibly. We believe everything we're told, and accept illness and over-priced drugs as just a part of life. When we're sick we want to feel better as quickly as possible. When drugs give us that relief we long for, we're willing to ignore the side effects and risks. Drug companies know that about us. It's what enables them to take advantage of us. They're hoping that we stay dependent on their products because we're less likely to ask questions when we really need something.

It's time we realize just how under the influence we really are.

[23]

What Does the FDA Really Do?

Most people assume that the FDA actually test and study products and that couldn't be more wrong.

The FDA is responsible for regulating the safety of all domestic and imported food and drug products. This includes assuring that foods are safe and sanitary, and that products like drugs, medical devices, supplements, and cosmetics are safe for use by the public.

What may surprise you is that the FDA is totally dependent on companies to provide data and evidence that prove safety. So the government depends on safety data that is provided by companies who want to get their product to market.

The FDA will only investigate and recall a product if the risk to the public outweighs the benefits. Meaning many people have to die, get sick or injured before the FDA steps in.

Oh, you should also know that many of the agents that work at the FDA use to work at the very companies the FDA is charged to regulate. Can you say serious conflict of interest!

But you're different from most parents. The fact that you're reading this book tells me that you're ready to learn the truth. Maybe you're tired of needing a drug just to get through the day. Maybe you hate the idea that some doctor or therapist is trying to put your kid on a drug that you know nothing about (chances are the so-called professional don't know much about it either). Perhaps you're like me and refuse to be manipulated by an industry that has chosen profits over people. The reason is not what's most important. Your decision to want better for you and your family is what matters most. In the coming chapters, I'll be giving you the facts and strategies you need to protect your family and to make important decisions, such as when to medicate and vaccinate.

The Healthcare Industry

More aptly named the Disease Care Industry; you don't have to be very enlightened to know that our healthcare system is a hot mess. The way it is set

[24]

up is the very reason why it is so poorly managed and so very ineffective. Consider this:

- Healthcare (a service) is provided by private companies (hospitals). Some of these companies identify as non-profits for legal purposes so that they can avoid paying taxes. The driving motivator behind these companies (hospitals) is longevity and growth in the form of profits. Growth outcomes, like most businesses, are measured by profits. These companies' annual reports don't measure success solely based on health outcomes of patients. They need to show profits and revenue.

- Private insurance companies have the majority of control. Their justification is that since they assume most of the risk, they get to dictate cost, care, treatment, duration, drugs, etc. The price of medical procedures that are not covered by your insurance are purposely inflated, making them completely unaffordable. Plus, with the Affordable Care Act we now we get fined for not having coverage. Americans are dependent upon health insurance. We don't make a fuss about this medical blackmail because we live in fear of losing coverage or not getting the treatment we need. Insurance companies are 100% about making money. They determine plans and coverage based on cost and need. Unhealthy people are more expensive to insure, but are typically life-long consumers of medical care. They keep hospitals and private insurers in business. This industry actually benefits from people being sick.

- Healthy people get penalized rather than rewarded. Insurance companies are able to offset the high cost of sick people by insuring healthy people. A healthy person may pay $4,000 in insurance premiums annually and only require about $250 in actual medical care. But wait, there's more! Healthy people also pay taxes to support Medi-Cal and Medicare programs for the elderly and those who can't afford insurance. Alternative medicine, which focuses on stimulating the body's natural abilities to heal itself, isn't even covered because there's very little money to be made off these services. So you have to pay for this type of care out of pocket. In essence, the healthier you are, the more you get screwed.

- Doctors are not sufficiently trained in prevention and nutrition. Historically, medical schools were funded by wealthy families like the

[25]

Carnegies who also had financial ties to drug companies. In exchange for funding, these families had a tremendous amount of influence on medical school curriculums. So it should come as no surprise that the primary focus of curricula was to train doctors how to diagnose disease and treat symptoms with drugs. Other schools of thought like holistic medicine or Chinese medicine were deemed as "quackery" or ancient folklore in order to eliminate competition. There is a considerable amount of money to be made off of people who think they don't have any options.

According to the 2014 *Commonwealth Fund Report*, a study which assesses healthcare services from a global perspective, the United States once again emerged as the world leader for the most expensive healthcare system. Not exactly the race you want to win. However, we are consistent. Compared to eleven other industrialized countries, the Unites States ranked last in areas of quality, efficiency, equity, access to services, and healthy lives. We die sooner and experience more illnesses than our peers in other countries. We consume more calories, use more prescription drugs and illicit drugs. Our children are more likely to be obese and less likely to practice safe sex. To sum it up, Americans are the unhealthiest, yet we pay the most money for the worst care and services.

At this point you might be wondering why you even bother. Maybe you feel powerless or overwhelmed by all this dismal information. I'm not sharing these facts to depress you. I am trying to light a fire underneath you because going numb and becoming a statistic is no way to live. You have options. Aside from moving to Europe, there are things you can do so that you don't become a victim of our crippled healthcare system. Stay with me because in chapter five you'll learn how to protect and be an advocate for your family's health.

Technology

Remember the days when all you had to worry about were the dangers that lurked outside your home? The biggest threats to your child's safety were the creepy guy who drove around asking kids to help him find his puppy, and the mean bullies at school. It almost makes you nostalgic for the days when you knew what to look out for. The list of identifiable threats was short and somewhat controllable. Plus, you could always find peace in knowing that your kids were safe when they were home. My, how things have changed.

It's an amazing time to be a kid. The internet and the advancements in technology have made the world smaller, communication faster, and information far more accessible. Technology has helped to create generations of kids and young adults who are more culturally sensitive, open-minded, and socially aware. It has sparked innovation and creativity in the minds of youths, giving them the idea that they truly can become what they want to be. Technology has become a powerful tool, yet at the same time it is a double-edged sword.

Internet-Related Challenges Facing Kids Today

> ➢ Becoming the victim of an online predator or bully

> ➢ Not knowing who to trust when sharing private information online

> ➢ Need to be liked and noticed makes them extremely vulnerable

> ➢ Self-worth becomes dependent on validation of others

> ➢ Use of adult technology makes them feel like adults

> ➢ Pressure to share sexually explicit photos or messages

> ➢ Inability to understand consequences of online behavior

> ➢ Lack of comprehension when it comes to online privacy, tracking, or permanency

> ➢ Can't recognize addictive behavior (adults struggle with this too)

> ➢ Life online can foster isolation and social anxiety

The challenge for parents, in regard to technology, is twofold. First is the development issue. Such a powerful tool requires a user to possess skills of reasoning, constraint, judgment, and emotional maturity. These skills often don't develop until late in adolescence. Hell, I know plenty of grown adults who are still trying to develop these skills.

We often associate good behavior, or the absence of bad behavior, as good judgment in kids. It's why most parents feel so comfortable giving phones and unsupervised internet access to their kids. In cases I've worked where kids have been victimized by someone they met online, parents were always shocked by their child's behavior. They say, "But we've talked about this" or "She's a good kid—I just can't believe this happened." I reply, "Your child probably can't believe it either." They never saw it coming because

[27]

developmentally they are vulnerable and limited. Their emotions are way stronger than their judgment.

Secondly, technology is totally outpacing you. It's a fully automated electric car and you're a diesel truck with no power-steering. You may not want to hear this, but you have got to take the time to get "user-friendly" when it comes to technology. I'm not saying you have to learn how to code and start hacking into servers but you are going to have to make some effort. Failure to do so will create this power shift in your home. When your child knows more than you do about the internet and apps, you are at their mercy. Some parents think it's cute that their kids have to teach them how to use stuff. I personally think it greatly limits your ability to protect your children. Chapter six is going to upgrade your knowledge about technology, enabling you to be a strong force against the dangers of the internet to your child.

Are you still with me? I'll assume you're nodding yes at this point. Well, get comfortable and let's dive in.

CH. 3 – THE COST OF CONVENIENCE

The family of ten-year-old Devin came to me as a referral. While I can't say who made the referral, I will tell you there were justifiable concerns about Devin's weight gain over the past year. Devin stood at about four feet, six inches tall, just slightly under the average height for a boy his age, but weighed nearly ninety-eight pounds. Now at that height, a child with a healthy body mass index (BMI) should weigh around eighty pounds. There were also concerns regarding changes in his behavior. It seemed that Devin went from being a cheerful, attentive student to a moody, easily-distracted little boy who was prone to toddler-like tantrums.

I had arranged to meet Devin and his mother Amy for a 10 a.m. home visit. I knew a crucial part to understanding these changes in Devin's weight and behavior was to see his home environment. When I knocked on the door that morning, I recognized a familiar voice coming from inside. It was Buzz Lightyear from the movie *Toy Story*. The TV was blaring, which meant I had to pound on the door for several minutes before I got somebody's attention. Once inside, it didn't take long to put the pieces together. I can remember the exact scene. Devin was seated on the floor about 2-3 feet away from the TV. He was laying on his stomach, still dressed in his pajamas. He was engrossed in the movie and never even bothered to look up when his mother introduced us. Every part of Devin's body could be described as chubby, but he was carrying the bulk of his weight in his belly. On the floor, directly in front of Devin was an open bag of Lay's potato chips and a bottle of Coke. Not a glass—a half-full liter bottle. And remember, it was only 10 a.m.!

Amy was completely transparent with me when she shared her story. She was going through a divorce from Devin's father and had been battling over custody issues for months. She also had a teenage daughter from a previous relationship that was doing poorly in school and engaging in some promiscuous sexual behavior. Needless to say, her cup runneth over with life challenges.

Amy explained that both her and Devin's father felt tremendous guilt over their divorce. She said that Devin started throwing tantrums like he was a toddler. He'd whine and beg for junk food, and if she told him "No," he'd throw a fit and start hitting walls and screaming. So she gave in and started buying salty snack foods and fast food because it seemed to pacify him. Amy explained that she knew the weight gain was not healthy, but didn't know how to fix it without sending him into a tail spin.

In most instances like this, a social worker would give Amy referrals to counseling and perhaps some educational guides on diabetes. A social worker might tell her that the state may intervene if Devin's condition worsened. I always felt like this wasn't enough. It was like seeing a parent hanging onto a cliff for dear life and then suggesting to them that they take a minute to read some helpful pamphlets. Plus, pointing a finger in their face only added to their guilt and stress.

Amy wasn't a bad parent—she was a good mom going through some fairly common life challenges. Instead of leaving her hanging, I tried to empower her and help her to restore some of that control she had lost. I educated her about the addictive qualities of processed foods as well as the effects these foods have on a child's developing brain and body. I also noted that too much TV was causing Devin to be sedentary. He would benefit both physically and emotionally by participating in outdoor group activities that could offer exercise, exposure to sunlight, and socialization. I explained that kids need boundaries and consequences, especially during time of transition and emotional uncertainty. The enforcement of rules can create a sense of security and reduce the possibility of a child manipulating parents during a time of discord. We also explored all her options for support in her community so she knew exactly where to turn when she needed guidance. When I left she looked relieved and hopeful–and not only because I was leaving. Devin's story isn't unique.

Over the years, I realized there's a very common thread that's weaving its way into the lives of many American families. As I mentioned earlier, food is the most powerful "drug" on the planet. The right kind in the right amount can keep us healthy and prolong our lives. The wrong kind in the wrong "dose" can kill us. As a parent, it is vitally important that you understand how to use food to nourish, protect, and heal your child. If you can implement this knowledge, it will have a profoundly positive impact on your child's health, both today and thirty years from now.

This is about saving your family. There are things you must know about the food industry in order to raise emotionally and physically healthy children. The news isn't pretty but remember, information is your friend. It may feel a little scary or hopeless at times, but it's even scarier to think of the price you pay for being passive and choosing to stay in the dark. My goal is to keep you informed so that your job as a parent gets easier, not harder. This is about you having peace and confidence in knowing that you are doing your best and teaching your children in the process.

What is the Food Industry?

For the purpose of this discussion, the term *food industry* includes all the growers, manufacturers and companies that make the food products we consume and feed to our families. The term *food* describes natural products that are raised (animals) or grown (produce and grain) and processed food products that are made in a lab and/or processed in a facility. When it comes to choosing foods, one of the biggest challenges that you'll face is knowing what to believe. There is an abundance of conflicting information when it comes to determining what's safe and what's not. It's best if we start by looking at some of the food facts that you may not know.

Are you aware that a good portion of our food comes from other countries? The United States imports 40 percent of its fruits and nuts; 20 percent of its fresh vegetables; and 80 percent of its seafood (Hamburg, n.d.). Thanks to budgetary cuts, the Food and Drug Administration (FDA) is only able to inspect about 2 percent of these imported foods. Not only are we totally unaware of how these foods are grown, manufactured, and tested, but these foods are at an even greater risk of contamination and degradation during shipment. This is why the National Institute of Health (NIH) stated that "Rightly or wrongly, imported food is held responsible for the greatest risk" to the foods we eat.

That's not to say that all the foods coming from other countries are bad. Many European countries have more stringent agricultural laws than the United States and use sustainable farming practices. Sustainable farming is the practice of using farming techniques that protect the environment as well as the health and welfare of people and animals. While the US agriculture industry agrees that there is a need for sustainable farming, everyone seems to have a difference of opinion as to how to implement it.

What we know with certainty is that the use of chemicals on our crops and with our livestock has polluted our entire food system. The book *Food Smart: Understanding Nutrition in the 21st Century* (Hunter 2009), provides consumers with valuable information on how our foods are raised and treated with chemicals.

For example, growth hormones accelerate the rate at which the meat of chicken and cows can get to market. They are fed a diet of corn and meat by-products from other animals which is unnatural. Since the corn is sprayed with pesticides, they ingest the pesticide residue which is stored in their fat cells. This unnatural diet causes distress to their digestive systems. They also get infections from living in cramped quarters, forced to stand in their own feces all day, with no room to move. To remedy this, they are given antibiotics.

Beef and poultry also get "chemical enhancements" to look more pleasing to the buyer's eye. Red dye is added to beef for that look of freshness, and saline is injected into chicken because we all like our chicken juicy and bloated.

Government Agencies
Cheat Sheet

Food and Drug Administration **(FDA)** – oversees the production, processing, packaging, storage and detainment of domestic and imported food

United States Department of Agriculture **(USDA)** – oversees the safety, wholesomeness, labeling, and proper packaging of domestic and foreign meats, poultry, eggs; regulates herbicide-tolerant crops

Environmental Protection Agency **(EPA)** – sets levels for pesticide residue in or on food, including animal feed; protects food supply from chemical and microbial contamination; develops national standards for drinking water systems

Center for Disease Control **(CDC)** – investigates food-related illnesses and determines standards for food borne illness prevention

National Institutes of Health **(NIH)** – part of Dept. of Health and Human Services; research on food-related pathogens and information important to determine what interventions necessary to improve public health and prevent disease

Let's not forget fish. Its chemical exposure happens in our oceans and lakes polluted with everything from mercury to chemical dumping from factories, to oil spills and even radiation from nuclear meltdowns.

Fruits and vegetables don't fare much better. The Environmental Working Group (EWG) reported in its *2013 Pesticide Data Report* that the United States Department of Agriculture (USDA) found evidence of 165 different pesticides in a sample of produce. Detectable residue was found on about 64 percent the sample despite some of the produce being washed and peeled. Surprisingly, the FDA, USDA, and CDC all agree that pesticides pose a serious threat to our health. Their politically correct response to the issue is that the health benefits of eating fresh fruits and vegetables outweigh the risk of ingesting pesticides. While this is true, it doesn't mean that we should just sit back and take our chances.

The truth is that we are constantly absorbing and ingesting chemicals from our produce, our meats, our environment, our drinking water, our medicines, and our household products. It all adds up to equal one very toxic human body. That is a problem.

In 2012, the American Academy of Pediatrics reported that children have "unique susceptibilities to [pesticide residues'] potential toxicity", citing research that linked pesticide exposures in early life and "pediatric cancers, decreased cognitive function, and behavioral problems" (Forman and Silverstein 2012). The organization strongly recommended that pediatric physicians provide parents with resources that inform them of the dangers of pesticides.

Has your pediatrician ever spoken to you about the dangers of pesticides?

Nutritionally-Challenged Produce

Our health is totally dependent on the quality of our food. Food should provide us with nutrients which are vital to our development, growth, energy, and ability to heal. Unfortunately, the nutritional value of our produce is not what it used to be. The Food and Agriculture Organization of the United Nations (FAO) explains that, "healthy soils supply the essential nutrients, water, oxygen and root support that are food-producing," noting that it can take 1,000 years to produce just .4 inches of healthy soil (2015).

[33]

Soil-grown foods are one of our greatest sources of minerals. This is especially important to note since our bodies can't make minerals; we must get them from food. The problem is that we are destroying healthy soil faster than we are replenishing it. Soil is depleted of its natural minerals and organic matter as a result of wind and water erosion, drought, irresponsible farming practices, overuse of chemicals, and waste dumping into landfills. As a result, the nutritional value of our foods has been on a steady decline over the past seventy years. The Nutrition Security Institute reminds us that, "without adequate nutrition, especially minerals, research has shown that people develop chronic health conditions" (Marler and Wallin, 2006).

It's no coincidence that our food has diminished in nutritional value at the same time that farming has morphed into one of the most powerful, privately owned social programs in the country. How can it be a social program and privately owned, you ask? Farmers basically receive welfare. That's right. The government subsidizes farming. In simple terms, the government gives farmers financial aid in the form of cash grants or tax breaks to promote production and support farming. It's much like how the government gives financial aid to parents to promote stability and support families.

These farm subsidies also support farms owned by giant corporations. Yes, those same corporations that want limited government regulations are receiving a form of social welfare. Wondering where the money comes from to pay these farming subsidies? An article in *The Economist*, entitled "Milking Taxpayers," reported that, "American farm subsidies are egregiously expensive, harvesting $20 billion a year from taxpayers' pockets. Most of the money goes to big, rich farmers producing staple commodities such as corn and soybeans in states such as Iowa" (2014).

We are essentially paying farmers to grow our food, and then paying for that food at increasing prices while our food decreases in quality. Even if a piece of fruit is nutrient-rich at the time of picking, it must endure days of travel before it winds up in our grocery bag. Produce is perishable, meaning it is subject to decay and loses nutrients with each passing day. It is one of the many reasons why people, especially children, develop nutritional deficiencies.

Nutritionally-Challenged Processed Foods

Perhaps the most important factor that contributes to the rise of nutritional deficiencies is our preference for processed foods. To better understand, let's examine what it means when the words, "enriched with vitamins," appear on the packaging of a food product. Basically, a food manufacturer takes a natural food like wheat in its whole grain form and processes it into a fine powder (flour). What happens during "processing" is that the wheat grain is stripped of its coating, fibrous content, proteins and essential oils, to the extent that is loses much of its natural nutrients. Even worse is that manufacturers often use chemicals to bleach this powder to produce white flour!

The manufacturer now has flour that is used in thousands of different food products, but really offers no nutritional value. So what do they do? They add synthetic vitamins and minerals to the flour and call it "enriched." The problem is that it can be difficult for the human body to absorb synthetic vitamins and minerals, unlike naturally occurring nutrients that are easily recognized by the body.

Processed food is loaded with chemicals like additives, dyes, preservatives and synthetic flavorings. So when you eat highly processed foods, you are essentially eating food with little or no nutritional value. However, you are getting plenty of chemicals, hidden sugars, salts, and fats.

Why would companies intentionally remove all the nutrition from food? Well, manufacturers were excited by the idea that they could increase the shelf life of a food and enhance its flavor and appearance by adding chemicals. No one was too concerned about the long term effects of this experiment. That is until studies started to reveal the link between consumption of food additives and health conditions like allergies, ADHD, skin abnormalities, infertility, depression, migraines, and memory decline. See, we don't just consume these chemicals and then eliminate them in our waste. The chemicals actually get stored in our cells…for a very, very long time. Don't believe me? Ever wonder how people can be checked for past drug use with a hair follicle test? These toxic substances don't disappear; they stay in us and cause us great harm.

Genetically Altered Foods

Once scientists discovered how to give eternal shelf-life to food products, it seemed that creating "super foods" was the next logical step. The term "super foods" is used to describe man-made plant and animal varieties that can withstand the natural threats of pests and disease. Perhaps you have heard about genetically modified organisms (GMOs). Unless you've been in a coma for the past ten years, you have probably heard a little or a lot about this new species of foods. GMOs have the potential to radically change the concept of food as we know it. I can't stress how important it is for you to understand what genetically modified foods are and how they will impact the health and wellness of your family.

Genetically modified organisms are plants grown from genetically altered seeds. This involves the practice of taking genes from one species and inserting them into another species in order to get a desired trait. Plant seeds can be

[35]

spliced with the DNA from other plants, viruses, animals, and even humans. Basically, scientists are altering the natural genetic coding of fruits and vegetables. This is very similar to the science behind vaccinations. In the same way you have your child injected with a small dose of a virus; your food is getting injected with small doses of viruses and pesticides. Mmm, yummy!

You'll hear this science referred to as "genetically altered foods," "transgenic," or "biotech foods." The goal is to create a new species of foods (that companies patent and own, of course) that are indestructible to viruses, bacteria, and pests, resulting in a higher crop yield. The idea is that more food will help us feed more people. These biotech or agrichemical companies promise this could be the solution to eradicate hunger throughout the world. This is bold claim that has no supporting evidence. Not to mention, that we already grow enough food to eradicate hunger worldwide. Our only obstacle is the fact that global shortages and pandemics are profitable and greed seems to always take precedence (Druker, 2004).

This is not a new science. In fact, certain GMO foods like corn, soy, sugar beets, and canola have been on the market since the 1990s. To date, the government is not requiring these foods to be labeled, making it difficult for you and I to really know what's in our food.

Why should you care about genetically modified foods? Imagine your family doctor hands you a bottle of mystery pills and says, "Give these to your child once a day as a nutrient supplement." He tells you most of it is made from fruit but there's some unknown genetic material from an unknown species in them as well. He reassures you the pills are safe but admits that they have never actually been tested on humans. He also casually mentions that the pills were made by the same company that makes pesticides. Would you give those pills to your child?

This is essentially what you are doing every time your child eats a genetically modified food. We should all be uncomfortable with the idea of consuming foods that have been chemically altered and produced in a lab without having the slightest idea of what's in them. Sure it looks and tastes like corn, but on a molecular DNA level, it is so much more.

There is no conclusive evidence to suggest these foods are safe. Research has been limited to short-term studies on lab animals. No one, not even the biotech companies, have any idea what the long-term effects of eating these foods will be. As you continue to gather information in order to make your own decisions, keep in mind the following data from the Institute for Responsible Technology's *GMO Myths and Truths Report 2014*.

- Sixty other countries require labeling of genetically modified foods.

- Cross-pollination has resulted in GMO seeds contaminating non-GMO crops.

- Many of the administrative decision makers at the FDA are former biotech and big agriculture employees.

- Biotech companies hold patents on these seeds giving them a monopoly on the food supply and control of the farming industry.

- These biotech companies have a history of creating products such as Roundup pesticide, bovine growth hormone (rBGH); both are linked to increased rates of cancer.

How Empowered Parents Choose Foods:

Empowered Parents Don't Rely on the Government for Protection

A study by the Federal Interagency Forum on the health and well-being of American children revealed that nearly half (forty-nine percent) of children consume diets that don't meet the basic recommendations made by the 2010 USDA Dietary Guidelines (2015). While it appears that kids are getting enough diary and meat, it was found that their diets were significantly lacking in greens, beans, whole grains, and fatty acids. This is one reason why it shouldn't come as a surprise that 1 eighteen percent of children and twenty-one percent of adolescents are obese.

The government is fully aware that the state of health for American youths is on the decline. It is constantly kicking out studies and findings to support what we can see all around us. What our government really needs to look into is the role it plays in promoting capitalism over the health and well-being of its people.

Doesn't it seem like a huge contradiction for our government to tell parents to feed children more greens and beans, while doing nothing to change the fact that most of the country's farmland is used to grow corn? In 2014, the United States grew 351 million metric tons of corn. The overwhelming

[39]

majority of that corn is either exported, fed to animals, or converted to ethanol (Robbins, 2001). Only a small portion of our land is used to grow produce for us to eat (4 million acres compared to the 56 million acres used to grow hay for livestock). The government also uses a considerable amount of taxpayer's money in the form of subsidies to aid these large corn farms.

Government regulatory agencies like the FDA are totally underfunded, which severely handicaps their ability to perform their duties. Food producers add thousands of chemicals to foods without FDA oversight or review. The FDA does not have the funds or technology to keep up with the invention of new chemical additives, and must rely on manufacturing companies for safety research. Instead, they focus primarily on reacting to known threats to public safety, like food contamination, rather than prevention, like inspecting facilities and testing chemicals. Basically, some of us have to be harmed or injured before agencies like the FDA and EPA step in. We also need to acknowledge the unethical practice of staffing the FDA with agents who previously worked for biotech companies. We are basically allowing a fox to guard the hen house.

President Obama signed the Food Safety Modernization Act into law on January 4, 2011. Its intent was to strengthen the FDA's ability to regulate and protect the public. Unfortunately, many states and private companies use the law to restrict private citizens from growing and selling produce from a home garden or farm. The reason for such intrusive power? To protect us from intentional and accidental food contamination. Hmm, I may be crazy, but I'm far more trusting of some lemons from my girlfriend's backyard then I am of a salad from Chipotle.

Government intervention always comes under the justification of "protecting us" and knowing what's best for us. I bet most of you didn't even know about this law. As with most government acts, this law was written and passed with no input and very little pushback from American citizens. We blindly trust and believe what the government tells us because—well, we've become dependent on the government to protect us.

The Average Diet

A survey of students in the 9th through 12 grades of both public and private school across the United States found that:

15% of students eat at least 3 serving of vegetable a day

28% drank at least one soda in the past 7 days while 11% drank soda three or more times a day

13% did not eat breakfast

Center for Disease Control. Youth Risk Behavior Surveillance - United States 2011. MMWR June 2012: (No. SS 61:4).

Dependence fosters compliance. Most people don't want to question something they don't really understand. We have completely forgotten that the government works for us, and should therefore have our best interests in mind. We also tend to ignore the fact that many politicians seem to be owned by industries and corporate interest.

As a result, the government has become rather inept at protecting us and defending our interests. I'm not suggesting that you rebel against the government, but I am strongly encouraging you to seek the truth. Don't just automatically assume that information is accurate or beneficial for you and your family just because it came from the government.

You'll see that I use government studies and reports for resources throughout this book. I also use independent studies and privately authored books as well.

When you have precious time to research a topic, a good practice to get into is to get your information from a diverse selection of resources. Look at journals, government websites, non-profit organizations, and books by qualified experts. If each of these sources are coming up with the same findings and information, that's a strong indicator that the information is credible and can be trusted.

Finding Quality Food Products

As mentioned previously, the nutritional value of food has declined significantly over the past seventy years. Without adequate nutrition, especially minerals, we know that people develop chronic health conditions. If you are serious about raising healthy children, you need to ensure that they eat healthy foods. To start, you must get rid of all the old myths and excuses that you've used in the past. Let's examine a few common ones.

Healthy Foods Don't Taste Good.
I've had clients tell me this for years. It's not that healthy food is bland. It's just that you and your kids are used to tasting synthetic chemicals known as flavoring. Like a connoisseur of fine wines, your kids have become accustomed to and addicted to these chemicals. For example, Flaming Hot Cheetos are a widely popular snack but they are not made with anything that even resembles cheese. There is nothing natural about the product, yet there are kids running around this country thinking that's what cheese should taste like. If you don't do much cooking at home or can't remember the last time you saw your child eat a vegetable, then making the transition to real food will be challenging at first. Your child will have to lose their cravings and basically reset their taste buds. But here's the good news; kids are far more flexible than

adults. I have yet to experience a situation where a child refused to eat and slowly withered away. They adjust.

My Kids Won't Eat It

I know from experience that what this really means is that as a parent, you don't like the food in question or you want to avoid the struggle of trying to get your kid to try something new. I have a good friend who swore her daughter hated fish. Then I later discovered that her daughter loved the fish sticks served at her school. When I jokingly questioned her about this, she admitted that she hated cooking fish and couldn't stand the smell it left in the house. Pediatricians and nutritionists both agree that a child typically needs 6-8 exposures to a new food before they'll start eating it. I'm also a huge proponent of hiding healthy foods in kids' favorites. For example: putting kale in smoothies; mixing pureed cauliflower in mashed potatoes; and adding ground-up veggies to casseroles and sauces. This is a great way to introduce them to new flavors.

It's Too Expensive

This is exactly what the makers of Flaming Hot Cheetos wants you to think. It is one of the greatest lies told to the American public. The biggest expenses when it comes to groceries tend to be dairy, meat, cereals, and snacks. These are the exact same products you should be trying to limit. Fresh produce, legumes, nuts/seeds, and whole grains are very affordable and a better source of nutrients. You can also buy them in bulk and really save some money.

Organic Produce is No Better Than Commercial Produce

Remember the *American Academy of Pediatrics* article stating that children have "unique susceptibilities" to pesticide residues from produce? I know there's so much confusing and misleading information out there about whether or not organic produce is worth the extra few cents. But the whole point to choosing organic is to reduce the risk of consuming pesticide residue. We live in such a toxic environment. We take toxic drugs, eat toxic foods, put toxins on our skin, drink toxins, and breathe them in all day, every day. Choosing organic is a great way for you and your child to reduce your toxic load.

We Eat Fairly Healthy Already

Despite having access to nutritious foods like fruits and veggies, Americans are still reaching for the potato chips. The *American Journal of Clinical Nutrition* found that 61% of the food we consume is highly processed and accounts for about 1,000 calories of our daily intake (Mendez, Wen Ng, and Popkin, 2015).

That means that more than half of the food we feed our bodies is a poor source of nutrients and energy. Our thousands of bodily functions that we take for granted (until we get sick) have to run on one-third of the nutrients they actually require.

If you want doctors and medicine and sick kids to be a thing of the past, you need to be honest about the effort you are making. This doesn't mean that you never get to eat pizza and cake again. What it means is that you recognize that these foods have little to no nutritional value and therefore should not be considered "food" but indulgences. Every time you give your kid a slice of pizza, you need to own the truth that you deprived them of their necessary nutrients. I know that seems harsh but this is the reality: pizza crust has no nutritional value and tomato sauce is not the same as eating a fresh tomato.

Start getting into the habit of acknowledging that "processed" (think pizza, cereal, hamburger helper, and macaroni and cheese) essentially means that all of the nutrients have been processed out. Strive to eat "farm to table," meaning: cook meals using foods that come straight from the earth or the farm, like fresh produce, and organic meats and eggs. Don't forget the fish!

Don't Get Suckered by Clever Marketing

Everything is not as it seems; especially when it comes to the processed food products that fill most grocery aisles. Companies spends a bunch of money to keep you confused and in the dark. Did you know that food and beverage companies spend most of their money on research, development, and marketing? The ingredients and components used for making so-called food products are relatively cheap. It's expensive, however, to hire chemists to create that special blend of chemical additives to addict consumers to a product.

> **DON'T BELIEVE WHAT YOU READ ON SOME LABELS**
>
> The **Center for Science in the Public Interest (CSPI)** works to expose fraudulent advertising and to put pressure on the FDA to take action. Some of their efforts include:
>
> Appeal to Gerber Graduates to stop claiming that it uses natural fruit juices in its snacks when high fructose corn syrup is the first ingredient listed.
>
> Appeal to stop General Mills Yoplait Yogurt from claiming that eating 3 servings of dairy a day helps to burn more fat which is a false claim.
>
> Appeal to Kellogg for its Eggo Nutri Grain Pancake claim that it was made from whole grains although it was primarily made from white flour.

[43]

The biggest checks get written for marketing expenses. Crafting commercials and packaging that play on our emotions cost a pretty penny. A product's success is heavily dependent on its marketing. Unfortunately, most consumers buy into it—hook, line, and sinker.

Most of the stuff printed on food labels is purely for marketing purposes. The goal of marketing is to grab your attention with either an image or words that touch on your emotions. Using words (or should I say, "manipulating" words) is a powerful marketing tool when it comes to selling food.

Certain words can make you feel as if you are buying a product that is good for you. Food labels can imply or suggest certain qualities about their product without it having to be true. Food manufacturers are far more concerned about what you THINK about a product versus the actual QUALITY of a product.

For example, there are a lot of nature-friendly adjectives thrown around these days. Terms like "All Natural" and "Free Range" make you feel like your groceries are coming straight from the farm.

Do Not Trust List	Terms Regulated by Guidelines
"All Natural"- products do not have to meet any guidelines or requirements to use this term	**"Organic"**- means that at least 95% of ingredients are organic; look for USDA logo
"Free Range"- amount of time animal outside is unregulated, could be outside for an hour and caged for 23 hours	**"Made with Organic Ingredients"**- means these products contain at least 70% organic ingredients
"Antibiotic or Hormone-Free" - hard to determine if claim is true and no one agency is monitoring	**"100% Organic"** - inspected, verified, and enforced; look for the USDA logo

Don't fall victim to these marketing tricks. Learning how to read nutrition labels on food packaging is one of the best ways to empower yourself as a consumer. Start getting yourself familiar with all of the alias names for harmful ingredients so that you'll recognize them immediately. For more information on how to read nutrition labels visit my blog at:
http://nourishedminds.com/learn-the-facts-about-nutrition-facts-labels/.

Producers of high-fructose corn syrup launched a global campaign to convince consumers that corn syrup is just the same as table sugar. They designed ads which depict soccer moms serving corn syrup juice boxes to convince you that their product is natural since it's made from corn. But don't be fooled. The corn they use is probably genetically modified and is so highly refined that it's completely chemically altered. Manufacturers try to cleverly disguise sugars found in processed foods under many different aliases and names. It doesn't matter what you call it because at the end of the day, it's still sugar and it's still harmful. Here are a few to keep watch for:

beet sugar	brown sugar	fruit juice	malt syrup
barley malt	glucose	maltose	maltodextrin
cane sugar	cane juice	molasses	raw sugar
caramel	grape sugar	dextran	sorbitol
carob sugar	corn syrup	dextrose	sucrose
date sugar	sugar	diastase	high-fr. corn syrup
fructose	lactose	yellow sugar	mannitol

Marketers tend to create campaigns targeted at moms and kids: moms tend to be the primary caretakers, cooks, and parents who are loading up the grocery cart; kids—well, because they're easy targets. Think about what most kids want: friends, to be cool, to fit in, to have special gifts or talents that give them recognition. Kids believe that products will connect them to others like their friends, icons, and heroes. Young children believe they can enhance their abilities simply by eating or drinking a certain food or beverage. This kind of mind voodoo works on us adults too.

Have you seen the *Got Milk* commercial with the cute little black girl sitting in a grocery store shopping cart who meets her future self? Her future self is homely, worn out and clearly depressed but musters the strength to encourage the little girl to drink some milk. The little girl takes several big gulps of liquid magic, and POOF!, her future self instantly becomes an attractive, muscular, gold medal-winning Olympian. Next we see the little girl's mom sweeping cartons of milk into the basket.

I'll give it to them…it's a funny commercial. But the funniest part is the fact that sixty-five percent of Americans can't digest the lactose in milk after infancy.

According to the *National Institute of Health*, lactose intolerance is most common in people of African descent—as well as people of East Asian, Arab, Jewish, Greek, and Italian decent. Hopefully that little girl's mom is up for all the late night tummy aches. Then again, maybe all that Olympic training will help to ease her gas and bloating.

[45]

I can't end this section without asking this, "Why do we care what celebrities and sports figures are eating and drinking?" Why would you take a recommendation from someone who has no expert knowledge and is paid to promote a product? It has nothing to do with the quality of the product.

Marketers know you want to be like them. Drinking the same brand of soda is about as close as you'll ever get. Remember, celebrities are paid to promote these products and then probably never use them again. I'm even willing to bet that some of them refuse to even swallow the products. Celebrity endorsements are blatant attempts at manipulating us into thinking we'll be a part of the "it" crowd by purchasing their products. You're way too smart for that, so don't give these companies your hard-earned dollars.

Shop Smarter

Your best bet is to do your homework and be your own consumer advocate. The good news is that when you're informed, you become a more confident consumer. You no longer have those feelings of uncertainty and powerlessness that typically cause you to make poor choices. You become an expert at spotting the clever marketing tricks and know how to use information to help you find brands and companies you can trust.

But not all companies are just about profits. There are many socially-conscious companies that are responding to the demands of consumers with quality products that are healthy and safe. With our support and buying power, we can help the companies that are pro-people to grow, while putting profit-hungry companies out of business.

I know that life can get busy and you may be feeling like it's time-consuming to monitor and regulate your child's diet. It may feel that way in the beginning but I promise you, it becomes easier once it becomes a

---

Know Your Brands

The following is a list of brands that practice sustainability, truth in marketing, transparency with ingredients, and/or are verified as being compliant with Non-GMO Project standards.

Braggs
Eden
Annie's Homegrown
Earth's Balance
Organic Valley
Nature's Path
Envirokidz
New Chapter
Pacific Natural Foods
Kettle Brands
Traditional Medicines
Pure
Nutiva
PJ's Organic
Bob's Red Mill
Lundberg Family Farms

Non-GMO Project Shopping Guide:
http://www.nongmoproject.org

[46]

habit. Remember, the goal isn't to change your life but to change the way you think and make decisions when it comes to the health of your family. Taking action can be as simple as choosing to avoid pesticides and genetically modified foods by purchasing true organic products whenever possible.

To keep costs down, stick to buying organic fruits and vegetables that otherwise have high levels of pesticide residue, aka "The Dirty Dozen." They include (in alphabetic order): apples, bell peppers, celery, cherries, grapes, lettuce, nectarines, peaches, pears, potatoes, spinach, strawberries, and potatoes.

You'll be fine buying regular commercial versions of produce with thick outer skins like bananas, avocadoes, melons and oranges. If you can't afford the additional cost or don't live in an area that offers organic versions, then try to purchase from small local farmers or get your produce from friends, family or neighbors who have fruit trees and gardens. Better yet, try growing your own!

Support Legislation That Requires Food Labeling

It's simple. You deserve to know the ingredients in your food. You have a right to know. If a company doesn't want to tell you what they are putting in your food, then why should you continue to buy their products? You are in control—not them. Spend your money on products made by companies you can trust and who are willing to be transparent when it comes to how they make your food.

Grocer associations and food manufacturing companies spend millions of dollars lobbying against legislation that would require them to be more transparent. That's how proposed laws for labeling of genetically modified foods were defeated in California and Washington. They resorted to using their worn-out fear tactic of claiming that the additional cost would be passed along to the consumer. Sadly, it worked. People got scared and worried that they would not be able to afford their box of ding-dongs and voted against the right to know.

I see truth labeling as a win/win situation for consumers. First of all, if you are a company that produces and packages good quality food, why wouldn't you want your customers to know what's in it? This is a great way to develop trust and create a lifetime customer. When a company refuses to list its ingredients, it's like that guy you meet on the internet that refuses to meet in person...you just know they're hiding something.

Let's even play the Game of Fears and say that food companies have to hike up their prices in order to print new labels and save their profits. The end result would be that you can no longer afford a food that is keeping you overweight, depressed, and unhealthy. Buying processed foods would no longer be in your budget so you would have to start eating more readily available fruits and vegetables. Companies pricing you out of their crappy products could be the best thing that ever happened to you. Labeling is your friend.

Collectively, we need to stop supporting companies that put profits before people, and demand action from a government that we put into power. Don't ever think for one minute that we are powerless against these companies and have no choice but to eat what they give us. We are consumers. We control the flow of money by what we buy and more importantly, by what we don't buy. Know what's in your food and question everything that poses a threat to the health and safety of your family. A great way to advocate for your family is to contact the members of Congress who represent your state and let them know what's on your mind. We elect them to represent our interest. The only way they'll know our concerns is if we tell them. You can find your representatives and state senator at www.congress.gov/members. Just click on your state and then the contact link to send them a form letter.

Important Nutrients for School Age Children (ages 4-11)

Allergies –The most common food allergies include milk, wheat, eggs, peanuts, soy and shellfish. I also encourage you to be on the look-out for food sensitivities in your child. Food sensitivities can cause subtle symptoms that may persist and appear to be totally unrelated to a specific food.

Some common allergy symptoms that can be the result of a sensitivity to certain foods include gas, stomach ache, diarrhea, earaches, ear infections, irritability, and dark circles under the eyes.

Development – Essential fatty acids (in the form of DHA, GLA, and EPA) are vital nutrients for brain development. They help to promote not only development, but learning comprehension and mood stabilization. Fat cells make up a good majority of brain matter which is why delays and learning disabilities are being linked to fatty acid deficiencies. Be sure your child is getting plenty of fish, seeds, and nuts in their diet or supplement their diet with an Omega 3 fish oil supplement made from wild caught fish.

Children of this age are undergoing a constant and rapid pace of physical development. Growth requires a significant source of energy from carbohydrate and protein for the development and maintenance of body tissues. Whole grains like oats and brown rice are good sources of carbohydrates while lean chicken, fish, beans, lentils, eggs and nuts/seeds are good sources of proteins.

Immune Support – Wherever there are groups of children, there are bound to be germs a plenty. Schools can be petri dishes and really put your child's immune system to the test. Try not to worry so much about your child getting sick. I know that's easier said than done but there is a benefit to being exposed to germs. A child's immune system is not like that of an adult's. It needs to learn how to identify and attack foreign invaders. The more practice it gets, the better it gets at its job. You can help to strengthen your child's immune system by adding foods rich in vitamin C (oranges, lemons, lime juice, broccoli, berries) and zinc (chicken, beans, almonds, pumpkin seeds, crab).

Important Nutrients for Tweens & Teens (ages 12-18)

Physical activity helps tweens and teens to grow bone and muscle tissue, and helps to promote healthy brain function and stabilize moods. All this work requires a considerable amount of energy and a regular supply of nutrients to nourish the body.

Keep in mind that your teen has a higher likelihood of developing deficiencies if they experience high levels of stress, routinely take medications, or refuse to eat certain foods like fish and vegetables.

Signs of deficiencies – Although mood swings and irritability are natural responses to fluctuating hormonal changes, they can also be directly related to nutritional deficiencies. Irritability, fatigue, or poor memory could be signs of **vitamin B** deficiencies. A **calcium** deficiency may show in the form of irritability or frequent muscle cramps; while signs of low **magnesium** levels include constipation, muscle cramps, depression, irritability, nervousness, and hyperactivity. Low levels of **vitamin D** may cause symptoms of mood swings, and can be a contributing factor in hormonal imbalances.

Consider these supplements:

Multi-vitamin –This supplement will provide your teen with a spectrum of vital nutrients to include all the B vitamins; small complimentary amounts of vitamins A, C, and E.

Vitamin D – Helps to support the immune system, stabilize moods, and maintain blood sugar levels.

Omega-3s – Omega-3 is an essential fatty acid and is essential for brain development and mood stabilization. Research shows that some learning disabilities can be linked to omega-3 deficiencies.

Calcium and Magnesium – Good sources of calcium include green vegetables, and organic yogurt while good sources of magnesium include bananas and whole grains. If your teen doesn't eat many green vegetables and is active in sports, they may need to supplement their diet. You will find these two minerals are often packaged together into one supplement because they work best when paired. Calcium and magnesium are needed for bone growth and density, good cardiovascular health and the production of hormones.

CH. 4 – THERE'S A PILL FOR THAT

I used to call 3 p.m. the "witching hour." Generally, my work days were quiet aside from the monotonous hum of the air conditioning and my daily meetings with staff and clients. But all that changed when the clock struck three.

You could hear their screams before the school bus even had a chance to grind its way into first gear and roll out the driveway. A quick click of the security locks on the front door, and then the entire facility would be filled with a symphony of high-pitched shrieking, skidding sneakers, and the thud of backpacks being flung down the hallway. It was madness, and for some strange reason I loved it; except for one particular day.

Back then, I was the manager of a residential treatment program that offered counseling and supportive services to families. It was a place where mothers and their children lived in an open community environment while they pieced their lives back together. My main duties were to make sure the program ran smoothly and to put out all fires. In recovery, there's always fires. Counseling and coaching those women was the best part of my job. I truly admired their courage and strength. Many of them were dealing with issues of depression, anxiety, and addiction, in addition to the typical challenges of being a parent. It was like fighting two battles at the same time.

[51]

When the kids arrived home from school, I would make my way into the common areas to do a brief emotional check-in with the families. Most days went well. This particular day did not. The scene was not unusual; an exasperated mother standing over her six-year-old daughter, barking orders for her to get off the floor. Meanwhile Clarissa, her daughter, was flailing on the floor engaged in a full-blown meltdown. I mean she was truly out of control. She was kicking chairs, throwing DVDs, and alternated between growling and screaming. When she got tired of kicking, she rolled onto her stomach and grabbed at the other children's feet who had stopped to watch the drama unfold. Every time her mother went to grab her, Clarissa would snap at her like a turtle. Or she'd do that thing where she arched her back and stiffened her legs so her mother couldn't pick her up. All the while, she kept repeating the same indecipherable rant.

Thankfully, years of this type of work had equipped me with a Zen-like ability to remain calm during emotionally-charged situations. Plus, I knew that getting angry with an angry child almost always ends in disaster. After dispersing the crowd of lookie-loos, I coached the mother through the process of managing her child's behavior. It took over thirty minutes before Clarissa calmed down. She eventually passed out from pure exhaustion. Then it took an additional thirty minutes for me to help the mother settle her frayed nerves.

Are you curious as to what had triggered this explosive meltdown? Well, when Clarissa had stopped crying and trying to fight her mom, I asked her why she was so angry. Her exact words were, "I want my Hot Cheetos and Dr. Pepper." Yep. This whole ordeal was triggered by a synthetic cheese product and caffeine. What I discovered later was that Clarrisa's mom had been using these after-school treats as leverage to get Clarissa to behave. On the day of the meltdown, the mom didn't have time to get the treats, which resulted in Clarissa losing her six-year-old mind.

News of the incident was reported to the behavioral therapist that had been seeing Clarissa weekly for the past three months. The therapist showed up in my office at the end of that day to share her concerns about Clarissa possibly having oppositional defiant disorder. She thought the six-year-old needed medication.

I have found myself faced with this dilemma more times than I care to remember. You should know that I am not a fan of giving psychoactive drugs to children. In the case of Clarissa, I fought the entire treatment team to postpone putting her on medication. My personal and professional opinion is that drugs are a last resort, especially when it comes to children. I also didn't believe that Clarissa had a mental health disorder. I felt that she lacked coping skills and suspected she had an addiction to sugar and caffeine. These substances act very similar to drugs in the developing body of a child. As mind-altering chemicals, they can cause behavioral shifts in children and impair normal brain function. When kids come down from the influence of sugar and caffeine, they experience withdrawals much like when an adult is withdrawing off of drugs.

With the mom's patience and the trust of my team members, we were eventually able to wean Clarissa off of foods and sodas that were chemically triggering her behaviors. She also started working with the therapist on coping with extreme emotions like anger and frustration. She still got angry and had tantrums but they were infrequent and much more manageable. Clarrisa's mom was also able to admit that she had emotionally detached from her daughter and used material things as a way to demonstrate her love. Clarrisa's behavior was a quick and effective way to get the attention she desperately wanted from her mom. It didn't matter that it was negative attention. When you're starving, you'll eat whatever is given to you.

Unfortunately, the type of treatment Clarissa received is rarely experience by children who present similar behaviors. The truth is that most doctors, therapists, and psychiatrists have very little understanding of the relationship between diet and mental health. As clinicians we are trained to treat with talk-therapy or drugs or a combination of both. There is no training on how to determine if a behavior is rooted in a nutritional deficiency, a toxicity, or a breakdown in one or more of the body's systems; the first places we should all be looking when it comes to treating physical and mental health problems.

Drugs don't even cure what ails us. They only mask symptoms or offer temporary relief. Aleve doesn't cure headaches, and vaccinations don't give us lifetime immunity (more on this in chapter 5).

How Did We Become So Dependent?

The answer to this question is twofold. First we must accept the fact that we don't like to suffer or feel any discomfort. It's as if we believe that it's more natural to be pain-free. We've convinced ourselves that the absence of pain and discomfort is health, and that's not necessarily true.

Our bodies are designed with an internal alert system to aid us in maintaining balance and wellness in the body. Think of it like the dashboard in your car. Nowadays, our cars' mechanisms are computerized. When they need something like an oil change, new battery, or more fuel, they tell us. A little red fuel pump icon or the word "oil" will light up, alerting you to take some action. This alert system is built into the car as a way to help you keep your car in good working condition.

Well, the human body has a very similar system, except our dashboard alerts come in the form of symptoms like pain, discomfort, or illness. The fact that your body is doing what it is designed to do is a healthy response. Try not to think of health as the absence of pain, but instead think of it in terms of functionality. For example, if you have a cold and you're constantly sneezing or coughing up phlegm; that is your body's healthy response and attempt to remove the infection from the body.

Too often we medicate these symptoms and think only of getting relief. The symptom gets masked but the underlying health issue still exist. We've conned ourselves into thinking that medicines cure us when in reality it is the body that cures itself. Medicines can suppress or stop the immune system from doing its job. When given the right support, the immune system is more than capable of destroying foreign invaders and restoring balance in the body. It's the real hero.

Our dependence has also steadily increased over the years, thanks to the brainwashing tactics of the pharmaceutical industry. Around the mid-1900s, a marriage took place that would change the lives of Americans forever: for good and for bad.

In 1951, Congress passed a law requiring consumers to obtain a prescription from their physician in order to purchase certain drugs. Prior to this law, people could purchase drugs, tinctures, and remedies directly from salesmen or a pharma (predecessor to pharmacist) who worked out of retail shops. Once the law went into effect, patients were required to first see a physician. This piece of legislation bound physicians and drug makers in a relationship that would become stronger and more dependent over the years.

Around the same time, wealthy tycoons like Carnegie and Rockefeller recognized the financial opportunities of marketing new medicines. They created foundations that provided the funding to start several of the country's prestige medical schools. As the primary investors, these industry moguls had a tremendous influence over the curriculum and training of medical students. They saw the potential for profits by training doctors how to treat patients with drugs and new innovative and expensive procedures. As a result, medical curriculum focused on classifying symptoms in order to treat them with drugs. Natural and ancient healing practices were deemed as "quackery" while medicine was touted as lifesaving. Thus began the marriage of capitalism and medicine.

It was easy to convince people that they needed medicine because the fact is that medicine is lifesaving. I said it before and I'll say it again: medicine is truly one of man's greatest accomplishments. But too much of a good thing is not only harmful; in the case of medicine, it has the potential to be deadly. The medical and pharmaceutical industries have managed to convince us that medicine is not just for emergencies, but that we actually need it to function from day to day. We are constantly being told that we are broken and that only

[54]

a particular drug can fix us. We've come to accept our dependence on drugs, so much so that we'll pay ridiculously inflated prices to get what we need. Dr. Richard Deyo and Donald Patrick, PhD, authors of the book, *Hope or Hype: The Obsession with Medical Advances and the High Cost of False Promises*, explain how pharmaceutical companies are able to charge such high prices because they know consumers lack the information and expertise to determine the effectiveness of a drug: "Anti-inflammatories and statins all work about the same but have different prices and different side effects." They point out that most consumers are totally unaware of less-expensive generic versions because we only know what our doctors tell us, and doctors get all their information from pharmaceutical reps.

What Drug Commercials Don't Tell Us

What these commercials fail to share with consumers is the information regarding success rates, failure rates, how the drug works, who did the research, and who funded the research. Instead they report misleading research findings. For example, a company may claim that a new drug reduces the risk by 50 percent. What we don't realize is that the original risk was 2 percent and the new drug reduced it to a 1 percent. Sounds great when a professional announcer reports it over whimsical animation, but not very impressive when you know the numbers.

There's another way that these drug companies manage to get into our pockets. Much of the research that goes into new drugs is funded by the National Institutes of Health, which is funded by—guess who—taxpayers. Then our government turns around and gives these companies patents on drugs, allowing them to have a monopoly on the product for up to twenty years.

I know it may seem like I'm painting a picture of a government that is working against us, but that is not my intent. The whole point is for us to take off our blinders so we can see the truth. It's the only way we can become empowered and make our government work for us.

Trending Drugs

Direct-to-consumer marketing has made it so that we can't watch TV or open a magazine without seeing a drug advertisement. Worldwide, the practice of showing advertisements for drugs on TV is not common. In fact, the United States is only one of two developed countries (New Zealand is the other) where the trend of direct-to-consumer marketing is permissible. According to a report

[55]

in the *Annals of Family Medicine* (Mackey and Liang, 2015), critics of direct-to-consumer marketing believe that the focus is put on the benefits of a drug while the harmful risks and increased likelihood of misdiagnosing and faulty prescribing are practically ignored.

By law, commercials are required to inform you about the possible side effects, but they never explain that their findings are solely based on clinical trials. Participants in clinical trials must meet very stringent requirements (known as controls) which don't make them good representations of the general public. That's why some of these drugs get approved, go to market, and cause catastrophic harm to thousands of innocent people seeking relief.

Like in the case of Vioxx. If you don't remember or never heard about it, Vioxx was anti-inflammatory medication prescribed to over 20 million patients. Over a period of more than two years, reports surfaced that the drug increased the risk of heart attacks and strokes. Yet the drug's marketer, Merck & Co., dragged their feet in taking it off the market, resulting in thousands more victims of its negligence. It was eventually taken off the market and became the largest drug recall to ever take place in this country.

Perhaps the most controversial growing trend is the practice of prescribing powerful, psycho-active drugs to children. Over-the-counter medications for physical ailments, and infection-fighting drugs like antibiotics and vaccinations have been used to treat children for hundreds of years.

It used to be rare and considered unsafe to give children mind-altering drugs. But that all changed about five decades ago. The practice of giving psychoactive medications to kids really began with FDA approval of Ritalin in 1961. By the mid-1980s, the number of kids taking Ritalin to manage behavioral problems rose to one million. Today, Adderall is the new Ritalin.

DRUG RECALLS

Here are a few other commonly used drugs that were eventually recalled after years of being in use.

ACCUTANE – for acne
In use for 27 years; increased risk of birth defects, miscarriages and pre-mature births in pregnant women.

CYLERT – for ADHD/ADD
In use for 30 years; caused liver toxicity/damage

REDUX aka Fen-Phen
Used as an appetite suppressant
In use 1 year; caused heart valve disease

DARVOCET – pain reliever
In use for 55 years; caused serious toxicity to the heart and death

Using Drugs to Treat Behavioral and Psychological Disorders in Children

In chapter six, we'll address the issue of using drugs to treat health conditions, but for now, I want to focus specifically on the risks and benefits of psychoactive medicines to children's health.

We have come far in our understanding of the body and disease, but we are nowhere near that level of comprehension when it comes to brain dysfunction. It's such a complex organ, and science doesn't have a clue how synthetic chemicals can alter our brains.

For years, those in the field of mental health (therapists, psychiatrists, and psychologists) have tried to make the treatment of mental health resemble that of physical health, more of an exact science. In effort to increase the consistency of diagnosing, the American Psychiatric Association adopted a system of classification. Disorders were identified and categorized based on symptoms with distinct criteria for diagnosing. This information was compiled into a manual known as the *Diagnostic and Statistical Manual of Mental Disorders,* or the DSM. To date, it is in its fifth edition (the revisions and creation of new disorders never cease to end) and has become the foundation for all mental health treatment. It is to mental health what the bible is to Christianity.

Originally this manual was intended for diagnosing and assessing disorders in adults. The signs and symptoms were all described in terms that applied to adults. Part of the standard criteria for diagnosing were age restrictions. Back when I was in graduate school, I was taught that best practices dictated that diagnostic criteria should only be applied to children over the age of five when assessing for behavioral disorders like attention deficit disorder (ADD), Attention deficit hyperactivity disorder (ADHD), and oppositional defiant disorder (ODD). These particular disorders were added to the DSM-IV (ADD appeared first in the DSM-III in 1980) specifically for children and adolescents to address what was considered childhood-related disorders.

It was rather unusual for a child to be diagnosed with a mood disorder, such as bipolar disorder, or a personality disorder, such as borderline personality disorder. The theory is that younger children are undergoing development changes that could easily be misinterpreted. The task of differentiating between normal development and symptoms of disorder can be tricky. This made perfect sense to me. The challenge became even more apparent when I started counseling school-age children.

I'll be honest; I was in way over my head when assigned to run a therapy group for nine-year-old students (all boys) diagnosed with ADHD. We met

[57]

once a week, after school, as a part of their educational support services through the school district.

Now I need you to imagine spending an hour, after school, with six nine-year-old boys with ADHD: all of them unwilling participants who thought group was "stupid." In the beginning it was BRUTAL! I was running the group like I had been trained, which was to have these boys sit in a circle (for an hour!) and talk about their feelings. That changed the day one of my clients threw a chair across the room out of pure frustration. What kid wouldn't be frustrated by having to spend their afterschool play time holed up in another classroom? Believe me, I felt their pain. I didn't even have ADHD, but wanted to start throwing chairs my damn self!

I decided to think outside of the box instead, so I started a basketball league with them. They got to help set the rules, draft players, and come up with team names. Now, you're probably wondering how basketball was going to help these kids with their ADHD. You may even be questioning my tactics at this point. I'll be the first to admit that I was young and just took a stab at it. My main motive behind choosing basketball was to physically wear them out so they had no energy to lift a chair. Plus, it was one of my favorite sports so I played along with them.

A few games into our little league and something magical started to happen. They calmed down. The game was allowing them to physically express their energy, but in a focused, positive way, but it did even more than that. They started creating plays and getting strategic, which required them to practice effective communication with one another. They would even high-five and cheer each other on. I noticed this kind of peer affirmation made them feel valued and helped to build their confidence.

There were scuffles, but even those incidents made for great opportunities to address impulsive behavior and practice self-restraint. I once overheard one of the boys who was the most aggressive of the group tell his teammate, "Hey, just walk away, it's not worth it." What! Those students have no idea how much they taught me. That experience was profound in my development as a counselor. I learned that children require very different types of interventions in comparison to adults. Children are less likely to learn by listening and far more likely to learn by doing. The same goes for behaviors; children are more likely to change a behavior when it's role modeled and practiced, compared to just being told what to do.

I discovered that when you combine learning with activity, it can make the mundane aspects of counseling become powerful tools for change. I'm not saying that all a child needs is a good game of basketball. What I am suggesting is that mental health practitioners should consider all options or even create new ones before resorting to medications.

Our use and dependence on drugs is strongly rooted in our instinct to avoid suffering. Much in the same way that no one wants to experience pain; we will gladly pop a pill to avoid negative emotions like anxiety and sadness, or even more intensified feelings like rage and compulsion. Drugs are powerful, fast-acting, and bring us relief. So it's no wonder that as a parent, you would consider giving your child medication to end their suffering. You should never feel guilty about wanting to find the fastest way to help your child. To help you make a decision that will also keep them safe, let's talk about both the benefits and risks that psychoactive medicines pose to children.

A small percentage of children and adolescents experience a transformation with the right medication. In cases where a child or adolescent has become a threat to themselves or the people around them, it is wise to consider drug intervention. It can bring relief to the child and also to family members who felt unsafe or lived in a constant state of fear. It can reduce violent or assaultive behavior, allowing a child or teen to remain in the home instead of having to be placed in residential treatment. With a proper treatment team in place, the child or adolescent can work with a therapist to develop the skills required to manage their disorder and a psychiatrist to manage the medication.

The American Psychological Association Working Group on Psychoactive Medications for Children and Adolescents found that psychosocial therapy or "talk" therapy is far safer than psychoactive drugs.

I have worked with many adolescents that experienced psychotic thoughts and behaviors. Sometimes these symptoms were the result of brain trauma and Antipsychotics, a form of mind-altering drugs, were the only things that helped them to quiet their minds long enough to do talk therapy. However, these kids make up a small percentage of the population. The majority of children who take psychoactive drugs experience either mild relief from symptoms or no relief at all.

Common Risk of Medicating Children

- Age, development, nutrition, stress, and toxins are all factors that can influence brain health and how drugs are broken down in a child's body. As a result, side-effects can range from mild allergic reaction and weight gain, to more serious side effects like seizures, suicidal thoughts, and death.

- Children can become dependent on a drug and adopt the belief that they need the drug to function. That's why psychoactive drugs are known as gateway drugs, meaning they often lead to the use or abuse of other prescription medications or illicit drugs.

- Psychoactive drugs only address the symptoms and don't actually cure, fix, treat, or heal the underlying cause of symptoms.

- Labels and the stigma of having to take medication can negatively influence a child's self-esteem, self-identity, and coping abilities.

Mental Health—More Art Than Science

Mental health disorders are believed to be the result of genetic expression or a chemical imbalance in the brain, although there is no actual science to support such theories. The assumption is that a chemical imbalance requires another chemical to restore balance, which is what leads people to believe that they need drugs to be "normal." Even in the absence of proof, we seem to accept the idea that drugs are our best remedy for these imbalances.

For reasons I can't explain, the behavioral sciences place little to no weight on the influence that diet and lifestyle has on an individual's mental health. I struggled with this as a mental health professional and I know I was not alone. Drugs are the preferred method of treatment because, sometimes, they work. Most people want instant relief instead of the work that comes with talk therapy; and to be frank, medicated clients can be easier to work with.

Besides the failure of our discipline to recognize the influence of diet and lifestyle, the other challenge that mental health professionals face is the subjective aspect of diagnosing conditions. Many years ago, I made the professional decision not to pursue my license as a clinical social worker. This went against all norms and confused my professional peers. I can't tell you how many times I was told that I needed to be licensed by the state in order to be considered credible and a professional therapist. Other licensed therapists explained to me that licensed therapists are held to a higher standard and governed by a code of ethics. I heard it all and it really made me feel pressure to conform and do what was expected of me.

Here's what I struggled with: The licensing exam is solely based on a therapist's ability to assess symptoms of mental health disorders and make an accurate diagnosis based on DSM criteria. They are then required to develop a treatment plan which identifies what type of action or therapeutic intervention they would take to treat the client.

[60]

Preparation for the exam requires extensive study of the different DSM disorder classifications (the most recent edition, DSM-5, lists over 300 disorders) and coding (this is a number system designed strictly for insurance billing purposes). In essence, a person who is good at taking tests and has a good understanding of the DSM can pass the test, get licensed, and go on to treat clients, but does that make them good at what they do?

I've had the opportunity to work with medical doctors, psychologists, psychiatrists, licensed clinical social workers (LSCWs), and marriage and family therapists (MFTs); all of which are required to be licensed or certified, depending on what state they live in. I've met some brilliant individuals; the kind where you wish you could absorb some of their wisdom just by being in close proximity. I've sat on treatment teams with some amazing professionals who showed such empathy and concern for their clients.

Yet at the same time, I have worked with licensed professionals who honestly have no business being in the business of counseling people. A running joke in the mental health industry is that some therapists become therapists because it's easier to help other people fix their lives than it is to fix their own.

The so called higher standards and code of ethics that licensed professionals are expected to adhere to don't amount to much if a person has a faulty character to begin with. Nor does it protect you from a therapist who is judgmental, hypocritical, racist, sexist, condescending, or suffering from their own mental health disorder. Not to say that you can't be a therapist with a mental health disorder, but you should damn well know how to manage it before you start counseling other people on how to manage theirs.

Perhaps the greatest challenge to this industry is the lack of supporting science. Unlike physical illness and disease of the body, mental health disorders don't have the support of science to link symptoms to disorders. Although the field of neuroscience is making progress, most of the theories on mental health have yet to be proven.

Mental health symptoms are self-reported and can't be measured. Physical symptoms like changes in blood pressure and tumors are measureable and can be tested, but there are no tests for insomnia or compulsive thoughts. The

Most Common Mental Health Disorders Diagnosed in Children

Behavioral Disorders:

Attention Deficit Hyperactivity Disorder

Depression

Autistic Spectrum Disorders

Anxiety Disorder

Post-Traumatic Stress Disorder

Obsessive Compulsive Disorder

Oppositional Defiant Disorder

[61]

art of diagnosis is rather subjective and is mostly based on the judgment and experience of the therapist.

For years, critics of the DSM have proclaimed that it's an unreliable diagnostic tool, and I tend to agree. I saw evidence of this during my years working as a clinical social worker. When I reviewed clients' mental health records, I was astounded by how many different diagnoses they had been given by different therapists over the years. What one therapist thought was bipolar disorder would six months later be diagnosed as anxiety disorder by a different therapist. Critics argue that you can have the same client seen by four different therapists who would come up with four different diagnoses.

I eventually chose to forego a license because I realized my greatest interest was not the practice of clinical therapy. My passion is in helping people to restore and maintain good mental and physical health with tools like nutrition, education, bodywork, and effective coaching techniques. Although I no longer practice psychotherapy, I firmly believe in its power and still use many of the interventions and therapeutic techniques in my coaching practice.

What matters most to me is what my clients think of my work. Many of them come to me after disappointing experiences with other professionals. I always stress that while education and credentials are good, it is the depth of a practitioner's experience and the quality of the partnership that matters most. I say partnership because as a coach, I make an investment in my client's success. It helps to build trust, accountability, and creates an environment where my clients feel safe and comfortable.

Over the years, my coaching practice has grown strictly based on word of mouth and my clientele has even included medical doctors and licensed therapists. I share all of this with you because it is so vitally important that you look beyond credentials and find a health professional who shares your concerns and beliefs, and is integrative in their approach to helping you and your family.

I highly recommend that you read the book, *Parenting the Whole Child*, by Scott M. Shannon, MD. Dr. Shannon is Assistant Clinical Professor of Psychiatry at the University of Colorado where he teaches an integrative and holistic approach to children's health. In his book he acknowledges that, "Our current medical system (from insurance companies to doctors) has become diagnosis oriented to the extreme. Once a diagnostic label is applied, it is often understood so rigidly that many potentially helpful treatment options are ignored (or disallowed by insurers), much to the detriment of the child in question."

Dr. Shannon speaks candidly about the risk of medicating children and his belief that a developing brain is easily influenced and far too complex to saturate with drugs. He exemplifies the less invasive, integrative approach of exploring safer treatment options before introducing a child's brain to psychoactive drugs.

"Poor diet is without a doubt one of the major reasons we're seeing such an incredible spike in the number of kids diagnosed with and medicated for mental and emotional disorders. Even drugs can't help kids when they are quite literally being starved of their mental and emotional health."

~ Dr. Scott Shannon, Parenting the Whole Child

How Empowered Parents Manage Mental Health

If you've made it this far with me then give yourself a pat on the back. You're a trooper because this chapter was pretty hardcore. You're also way ahead of the game. You now know more about the drug industry than most mental health professionals! I can say that because I used to be in the dark too.

When I was in graduate school, we were trained on the DSM but there were no classes or training on the holistic approach. The good news is that, I believe, that's changing. There are more and more professionals like me who are opting out of the traditional practice of treatment to adopt a safe, holistic service option for families.

You are the parent and that title gives you the responsibility and the right to make decisions that are in the best interest of your children. My job and the job of other service providers is to ensure that you have all the information you need to make informed, confident choices about your child's health care. Our support should be given without judgment, intimidation, pressure, or monetary motives.

Ultimately, you want to create a team of trusted, supportive, knowledgeable professionals who understand the importance of taking an integrative, holistic approach to health care. I know that fear and frustration can push you to make impulsive or panicky decisions, but try not to rush to action without thoughtful consideration of all your options.

Social & Developmental Challenges That Can Influence Your Child's Assessment and Treatment

- Young children lack the verbal skills to accurately describe their feelings and symptoms.

- Young children may not fully understand concepts of time and may have difficulties describing how often or how long they have been experiencing a symptom.

- Children are often influenced by their parents' thoughts/beliefs about the problem; this can have an impact on what they report to a counselor.

- Conditions like fear, hunger, and sleep deprivation can all greatly influence a child's behavior and statements.

- Understanding children takes time and patience; children with limited verbal skills may struggle to verbalize their thoughts and emotions. For the counselor, observation is a crucial aspect of the assessment.

- Kids don't always know what's wrong. Both children and teens may lack insight into their own thoughts and behaviors.

- Many drugs prescribed to children have only been tested on adults in clinical trials. This makes it problematic for physicians who have no scientific research to support their dosing decisions.

As parents, you don't need to create health in your children. It is already within them. Your job is to find supportive professionals who will help you to identify and remove barriers to health. Your children's minds and bodies will do the rest.

When symptoms appear...

➢ Refrain from going down the rabbit hole. Jumping to conclusions can make you feel like you don't have control and amplify your fears.

➢ Observe. Pay close attention to physical and mental signs of an underlying issue. Try to see if there is a pattern like irritability after eating certain foods or anxiety triggered by certain events. Document your observations over 1-2 months' time if you can.

➢ Have your child's diet properly assessed. Many mood and behavioral issues are rooted in malnourishment and deficiencies. Unfortunately, you may not be able to get this type of service from your general practitioner or a nutritionist. They may have a basic understanding of nutrition but lack advanced knowledge about the mind-nutrition connection. Consider seeking help from an integrative medicine practitioner, naturopathic physician, or a holistic nutritionist.

➢ Note any changes in your child's lifestyle or environment. This can be as simple as a change in cleaning supplies you use around the house to more stress-inducing changes like moving or loss of a friendship.

➢ Talk with your child about the behaviors and symptoms. Try to use the same words they use to describe their emotions and thoughts. The purpose of the talk is to comfort your child and also gain insight into the matter. Doing this when you're angry, frustrated, or giving consequences usually does not yield good results. Ask open-ended questions that aren't accusatory such as "Can you tell me what it feels like?" or "What's upsetting you right now?" or "What do you think would help you to feel better?" Asking question like "Why did you do that?" or "What's wrong with you?" will usually be met with an "I don't know."

When you believe it's time to seek mental health services...

➢ Your initial thought may be to seek treatment from your family doctor or general practitioner. I ask you to consider this—doctors specialize for a reason. You wouldn't go to the dentist for that suspicious mole on your back. Something as important as your child's mental health deserves specialized care. Review your insurance coverage and try to find a therapist or child psychologist for an assessment. You don't need to start off seeing a psychiatrist. If you decide later to try drug therapy, your therapist or psychologist will refer you.

➤ Focus your research on therapists who work exclusively or mainly with children.

➤ Confirm their education and experience, but more importantly, watch how they engage your child. Is there chemistry? Are they empathetic and encouraging? Does your child feel comfortable with the therapist? Are they answering your questions?

➤ For that first session, keep things light. Use this time for qualifying the therapist rather than going into your whole family history. This way it's easier for you to move on if you don't think it's a good fit. Plus, you don't want to put your child in the position of having to open up to all these new strangers. Just tell them a little about yourself and learn everything you can about them.

➤ If your therapist can't offer up at least three different mental health therapies to try (not including drugs) then look for another therapist. A good therapist is trained in a bevy of different treatment options.

➤ If you find a therapist you like, tell them you understand that labels and diagnoses are required for insurance coverage purposes, but that you'd rather they focus on specific challenges like impulsivity. Ask for a treatment plan that identifies goals for both you and your child. Be open to the reality that you may need to change some of your behaviors and beliefs about your child as well.

➤ Be confident and direct. Remember that you are the expert on your child. Your child needs you to be their advocate. Trust your gut. If something doesn't feel right and they are reaching for the prescription pad ten minutes into your visit, recognize that this is not who you need. Your child's emotional well-being deserves the highest quality of treatment.

When you've decided that your child needs medication...

➤ Be sure you have fully utilized all other treatment options.

- Find a psychiatrist that works with children and respects your concerns. If they start talking chemical imbalances and you see Pfizer logos on all their stuff, then thank them for their time and roll out! If they demonstrate transparency and acknowledge that psychiatry is more art than science, then you may have found yourself a winner.

- Never go off script. Give the medication exactly as directed. Remember, clinical drug trials determine dosing based on responses in adults. There is little to no research or standards for dosing children. Be assertive and tell your doctor you want to start with the lowest dose possible.

- Avoid trying new drugs that have been on the market less than three years. It is a well-kept secret in the pharmaceutical industry that medicines are rarely improved. Sometimes only one or two components of an old drug are changed and given a new name with a new promise. There is no scientifically conclusive data that any one drug is better than another. To play it safe, tell your doctor that you will only consider medicines that have been on the market for ten or more years.

- Ask for the generic version. These drugs are the same as name-brand. The only difference is that the drug-maker no longer holds a patent so other companies can access the ingredients to create cheaper versions that are just as effective.

- When discussing medications with your doctor, be sure to ask about: the result of clinical trials, how long the drug has been on market; the known side-effects; long-term effects; if it is addictive; if it can cause dependence; drug interactions; how long my child needs to take it; signs of adverse reactions that I should look for; what to do if my child has an adverse reaction; what to do if my child misses a dose.

- Tell your doctor that you'd prefer short-term drug treatment and would like to create a schedule that would eventually wean your child off the medication.

- Understand that medications deplete nutrients in the body so you will have to adjust your child's diet to increase their nutrient intake so that they don't develop deficiencies.

[69]

- Keep a copy of your child's prescription to ensure accuracy and for your medical records. If submitted electronically, request a paper copy.

- Be aware of signs and indicators that your teen is abusing their prescription medications. I have a great tip sheet at my website NourishedMinds.com.

Remember…Scientists Are Humans Just Like Us

We tend to view the scientists that create and test drugs as being these intellectually superior beings whom we are to believe because of their job title. But let's not forget that like many other professional, they went to school, studied, practiced, made mistakes, and gained expertise. Aside from their highly specialized education and training, they are normal people like us. They have feelings, doubts, opinions, and biases. They disagree with each other and sometimes they get it wrong. Some scientist succumb to the pressure of manipulating data, withholding findings, and embellishing reports.

It's also quite common for scientists to use general vague phrases to satisfy our questions, such as this drug or food "has not been proven harmful." What they are really saying is that either no one is studying the possible risks or there's not enough evidence to prove harm conclusively (which requires a lot of money and extensive research).

MENTAL HEALTH THERAPIES TO CONSIDER

THERAPIES	Focus & Benefit
ACUPUNCTURE	A practice based in ancient Chinese Medicine that uses needles and herbs to alleviate pain, headaches, anxiety, and depression. Acupuncture has been used as an effective form of treatment for thousands of years.
AROMATHERAPY	A gentle, non-toxic approach that uses essential oils and botanical herbs to relieve mental and emotional tension. These oil can be diffused into the air or applied topically. It is very useful in helping to calm and soothe young children and promotes relaxation and sleep in all ages.
ANIMAL–ASSISTED THERAPIES	A good body of research has found that a connection with animals, specifically dogs and horses, can help to bring about feelings of calmness, security, love, and positive energy. Animal-assisted therapy is especially beneficial for kids who struggle to open up or connect with others.
ART THERAPY	This approach can help kids express themselves through the creation of art, whether it's drawing, painting, sculpting, dancing, singing, or writing. This is really helpful with boys who struggle to express emotions because of gender or cultural beliefs.

[71]

MINDFULNESS MEDITATION & VISUALIZATION	While it can be difficult to get kids to sit still for long periods of time, studies found that even short moments of quieting the mind can help kids to develop self-control, self-calming skills, and reduce anxiety. Visualization helps kids to develop positive self-images and is a powerful tool to change their state of mind.
NEUROLINGUISTIC PROGRAMMING (NLP)	The focus of NLP is to reprogram faulty thinking and beliefs that are feeding into anxieties, self-doubt, low self-esteem, and feelings of depression. This approach is evidence based and is utilized to compliment other forms of therapy.
NUTRITION THERAPY	Looks to identify a causal relationship between diet and mental health. It can help to identify deficiencies, allergies, food sensitivities, and toxins that may be negatively influencing behavior, mood, and physical health.

Tools to Empower:

Med Watch Safety Alerts

Helps consumers to stay informed on current safety issues with drugs, medical devices, and medical procedures.
www.fda.gov/Safety/MedWatch/SafetyInformation/SafetyAlertsforHumanMed icalProducts/

Medication Guides
Provides consumers with information on comprehensive list of medications and the serious adverse side effects from these medications.
www.fda.gov/Drugs/DrugSafety/ucm085729.htm

New Pediatric Labeling Information Database
Comprehensive database of drugs that the FDA has approved for use with children; lists recent changes to labeling as well as findings from recent studies. This is a great resource to use if you have concerns about any medication prescribed to your child. Citing this information with the prescribing physician will help you to determine if your doctor is up-to-date on research findings.
www.accessdata.fda.gov/scripts/sda/sdNavigation.cfm?sd=labelingdatabase

Society for Developmental & Behavioral Pediatrics
Find a clinician in your community that specializes in developmental issues.
www.sdbp.org

American Board of Integrative Holistic Medicine
Find an integrative holistic physician in your community.
www.abihm.org/search-doctors

American Association of Naturopathic Physicians
Find a naturopathic physician in your community.
www.naturopathic.org/AF_MemberDirectory.asp?version=2

CH. 5 – THE GREAT DEBATE: VACCINES

A good friend of mine had received one of those alarming letters from her daughter's school. Apparently whooping cough was spreading on campus. Nothing close to being epidemic, but enough cases to warrant a notification. My otherwise calm friend typically wouldn't be worried, but her five-year-old daughter Cami had recently had the flu and was left with a persistent cough ever since. She decided to take Cami to see the pediatrician the following day. After an extended wait in a crowded lobby, they were escorted back into a kid-friendly examination room. My friend shared her concerns with her pediatrician but didn't want to come off as some paranoid mom. She said her doctor had a way of making her feel like she was a bad mom or over reactive. Without much questioning, my friend's pediatrician quickly dismissed the notion that Cami had whooping cough and gave her a prescription for antibiotics. I should note that the pediatrician did not perform a throat culture or any real diagnostic assessment to determine that antibiotics were necessary.

It's what her doctor did next that was shocking, and unfortunately all too common. Her pediatrician briefly reviewed Cami's chart and noticed that the child was not up to date on her immunizations. She told my friend that Cami was behind on her shots and chastised her a little for not having come in sooner (cue bad mom feeling). The pediatrician then proceeded to give Cami six vaccines!

When I heard this I was angry enough for the both of us. That pediatrician showed such negligence in her actions and my friend had every right to be upset. I won't even get into her bad bedside manners. Do you know why the pediatrician's decision to vaccinate Cami was poor judgment? It was crystal clear that Cami's immune system was weakened, as proof of her inability to fully recover from the flu and her persistent cough. Nor was whooping cough ruled out. I'm no MD but I do know that no one, especially children and pregnant women, should be given vaccinations if their immune system is compromised. This warning is noted on vaccine inserts and posted all over the CDC website. Every doctor should know this and they also have a responsibility to explain this risk to parents.

Our Goal

Before I get started, let's get clear about the intent of this chapter. I'm not trying to change your mind or steer you to my way of thinking. I will lay out a buffet of researched information so you can make an educated decision about what is best for you and your family, and I will offer up-to-date resources that can help you with decision-making. All I ask is that you take fear out of the choosing process. Drawing conclusions based on fear is how many people end up with misguided beliefs. You'll never find your truth if you only focus on the information that supports your current beliefs.

As an Empowered Parent, you will no longer create beliefs based on bad advice or information blindly accepted as truth. You have separated yourself from the mindless herd and now you feed off of truth and proof. So many people look for information that will prove them right rather than seeking information that will prove them smart. Don't be one of them. Keep an open mind…that's the only way that knowledge can get in.

Don't seek information just to support your beliefs. That's not learning. Seek information that elevates you to a higher level of understanding. That is real growth.

Hopefully by now, you understand the importance of asking questions. Even if it means you are questioning people with letters like "MD" behind their name. Doctors and scientists are human and prone to mistakes and faulty beliefs just like the rest of us. You should also continue to question my information and determine if you believe it to be credible and of benefit to you.

The vaccine debate is about your rights as a parent and the safety and effectiveness of vaccines. At the heart of this debate is the issue of freedom of choice and the right of a parent to protect their child. We'll discuss this more in the "Being Empowered When It Comes to Vaccines" section of this chapter but for now, let's talk about the safety and effectiveness of vaccines.

The Cliff Notes Version of the History of Vaccines

Infecting yourself with a disease to reduce the risk of being infected with a full blown version of that disease is not new medicine. A less sophisticated version known as inoculation was practiced in Asia as early as the 1600s. In an effort to combat the epidemic of smallpox, the pus from an infected person's active smallpox lesion was transferred to a non-infected person.

How, you ask? You can read all about it in the book, *Pox Americana: The Great Smallpox Epidemic of 1775-82* by Elizabeth Fenn. An incision would be made on the recipient's arm with a knife or scalpel and then the pus from the lesion would be transferred into the open cut. Seems rather medieval, right?

Well, not much has changed in four hundred years. We've gotten slightly more sophisticated in that we use needles instead of knives, and now we add a bunch of chemicals to the pus so the virus doesn't die from the effects of temperature and time.

What many believe to be the world's first vaccination was performed in 1796 by Edward Jenner, a country doctor in England. Derek Baxby explains in his book, *Smallpox Vaccine, Ahead of Its Time*, that not unlike the inoculations in Asia, Edward Jenner used the pus from cowpox on a milkmaid's hand and inoculated a young boy.

Jenner went on to become a celebrity. Kings embraced his new vaccine and used national campaigns to promote mass inoculations to demonstrate their commitment to the health of citizens.

A research article in *Annuals of Internal Medicine* noted that the British Parliament awarded Jenner over a million dollars for his great contribution to society (think early 19th century currency like land, gold, property). Vaccines eventually came to the US in the early 1800s around the same time that exploratory expeditions brought vaccines to other countries throughout the world.

Why did governments have an interest in vaccines? The fact is that people were getting sick and dying by the thousands. Outbreaks of highly contagious diseases such as smallpox, measles, diphtheria, and scarlet fever were widespread throughout England in the 1700s and travelled with the settlers to

America. It was smallpox that posed the greatest threat to the developing nation.

This disease was so powerful that some historians believe it was responsible for the demise of many historical empires. It plagued Europe and America for centuries. From the moment smallpox landed on American soil, it had a devastating effect of the population of settlers and was responsible for wiping out the indigenous natives. Even with the advent of the vaccine in the late 1700s, smallpox continued to threaten the health and lives of the American people.

Despite the availability of a vaccine, smallpox continued to spread during the 1800s and early 1900s. Poor working families didn't always have access to lifesaving medicines. Basic needs like, heat, clean water, detergents, fresh foods; all the things needed to stay healthy, were exclusive to the wealthy.

Working families struggled to afford such luxuries. Poorer neighborhoods lacked sanitation and became breeding grounds for disease. Chronic malnourishment made it very difficult for people to recover from illnesses. "It's a Hard Knock Life" wasn't just the theme song for orphans like Annie: thousands suffered as a result of the unequal distribution of wealth in the post-war Industrial Age.

If you truly want to understand the politics of vaccines, I highly recommend the book *State of Immunity* by James Colgrove. He does a much better job of explaining how the management of pandemic disease became a government matter. He also explained how the poor became viewed not as victims but as breeders of disease.

The author goes on to explain that outbreaks of diseases like smallpox almost exclusively originated in overcrowded immigrant populations where poor sanitation and lack of access to heat, clean water, and nutritious foods were the norm. This is why the first mandatory vaccine law was enacted in the United Stated in 1809.

The government and supporters of the vaccine saw a direct link between poverty and disease. So to them, it seemed logical that the poor should be vaccinated in order to manage and eventually eradicate the disease. Immigrant families and poor families were not only mandated to get the vaccine but were quarantined if they refused.

Despite protest by healthy citizens and appeals by the Anti-Vaccination League, the practice of mandated vaccines spread to employees of companies, college campuses, and eventually school children.

Timeline of When Common Vaccines Came Into Use

Pertussis (DTP)	Diphtheria	Tetanus	Polio	MMR
1902	1926	1938	1955	1960s

1953 – CDC recommends 16 doses of 4 vaccines against 2 diseases by age 6

1983 – CDC recommends 23 doses of 7 vaccines against 3 diseases by age 6

2013 – CDC recommends 49 doses of 14 vaccines against 14 diseases by age 6 and suggest that a child can receive up to 8 vaccines at a time despite the absence of evidence-based research findings that this is a safe practice.

The belief was that vaccines would eradicate disease. However, our current vaccine schedule suggests that this is not always the case. Sure, some diseases have basically become ancient history, but others persist to this day. Perhaps we need to be questioning if more vaccines are resulting in more protection and healthier children.

This country is very prevention-focused when it comes to vaccination against historical disease, yet when it comes to the greater risks of asthma, obesity, diabetes, and leukemia, we are more reactionary. Why is it that the government keeps adding more vaccines to the schedule, yet our children keep getting sicker?

Becoming Part of the Herd

You may have heard of the terms "herd immunity" or "community immunity". These terms are based on the belief that if a sufficient portion of the population has immunity to a disease through vaccination or prior illness, the disease is less likely to spread; even to those individuals who are not vaccinated.

The CDC has practiced on the basis of herd immunity for years. It is the theory that supports the vaccine industry's claim that vaccines are responsible for eradicating major disease among the general population. Under this

[79]

premise, those that choose not to have their children vaccinated do not pose a threat to the general population. Yet these claims and beliefs seem to raise more questions than they do answers.

Risky Business?

Vaccines are biologic agents, meaning that unlike chemical agents which are more stable, they can be compromised or altered at any point in production from lab to vial. When a vaccine is compromised it can cause infection instead of immunity.

I'm always astounded by people who put more thought into buying a car or a new cell phone than they put into the care of their body. I know people who will go online and research the different models and features. They'll do price comparisons, read consumer reports, consult Yelp, and ask friends and family; all before signing the dotted line.

If this applies to you, then pat yourself on the back. Way to go! Researching and educating yourself is the best way to go about making important decisions.

What about when it comes to what you put into your body? Are you giving your health the same due diligence? Why is it that most people will eat, drink, inhale, or inject things into their bodies that they know nothing about without question? We're all guilty of taking our health for granted. Our bodies just seem to run on autopilot, so we think very little about protecting them.

We know better. Sure we're living longer, but we're not necessarily living better. If you're serious about taking back control of your health and the health of your children, you have got to start treating your body like it's the only one you've got. That means getting educated about foods, environmental toxins, medicine, and yes…vaccines.

Your approach to protecting your body should be like that of a security guard. You're responsible for checking everything that gets in and on your body. To do that, you need to be able to answer these three important questions:

1. How will this benefit me or my child?
2. Is this potentially harmful to me or my child?
3. Do the benefits outweigh the potential harm?

Once you know the answers to these three questions, you'll know your decision. And this is exactly the same approach that we'll take in determining whether or not you want to use vaccines as a preventative measure.

I'm a huge fan of pro and con lists, so this next section will identify both the pros of vaccine use and the cons. More importantly, I will use this section to dispel some of the myths and fear mongering used by the media to influence how you think.

Effectiveness:

Pros

Vaccines have been used for hundreds of years to reduce the spread of disease. Advocates of vaccines are quick to note that vaccines were responsible for the eradication of smallpox. Unfortunately, there is no scientific evidence to support that vaccines were solely responsible for wiping out smallpox. What historical data shows us is that cases of smallpox were on the decline at the time that the vaccine was invented. Possibly the combined result of improved sanitation and advancements in healthcare were responsible. When vaccines came on the scene, they showed valid effectiveness at preventing the spread of disease in what were considered high risk population. This fact should not be undermined. Vaccines saved people's lives and we need to give credit where credit is due.

Thankfully, the online world of data is swimming with pro vaccine research that supports the effectiveness claim, but not all research is created equal. Remember what we've learned from earlier chapters that it's crucial to know who is behind the funding for research. If you are seeking the truth, then rule out any research or claims that were funded by the pharmaceutical industry. They are often biased, vague, and sometimes based on faulty research methods.

Instead review independent research by non-affiliated organizations or researchers. I've included a couple links to government funded organizations that post current reports and tend to have more accurate data. Even government research can be a slippery slope since the government is a major investor in the vaccine industry. So proceed with caution and questions.

Institute for Vaccine Safety
www.vaccinesafety.edu/Aboutus.htm

National Vaccine Advisory Committee
www.hhs.gov/nvpo/nvac/reports/index.html

Cons

Now let's talk about the information that doesn't get reported on the six o'clock news. This nugget of truth may surprise many of you because it is one of the best kept secrets of the vaccine industry. The fact is that vaccines do not always give you lifelong immunity from a disease. Originally, scientists thought they did but believe it or not, the scientists got it wrong (which by the way is how things are discovered in science...by trial and error). What we've learned is that a vaccine loses effectiveness over time, which is why most vaccines are now given in multiple doses spread out over time.

Vaccinations & Immunizations Are Not the Same

To be clear, vaccines are not immunizations. Immunization means that the body has developed immunity to something by natural means. For example, I got chicken pox at age 23. I was naturally immunized and now I'm immune from getting chicken pox again. Vaccinations are man-made compounds that are injected directly into the blood in order to mimic the natural process of immunization. However, what many people fail to realize is that they are temporary. Vaccinations don't always provide you with lifetime immunity.

So even if you get vaccinated, you are not completely protected from getting the disease years later. There are a couple other interesting facts about vaccination that you need to know. In some cases, after you receive a vaccination, you are contagious. Yep, you heard me. You are at a heightened risk of spreading the disease to other people. This risky period is called "shedding" and it's when you present with slight symptoms of the disease; enough to transfer the virus to another person. So in a non-intentional way, vaccines may also contribute to the spread of the disease.

But wait, there's more! Viruses like the flu often mutate over time which means that their DNA changes. When you hear doctors or scientist refer to a "strain," they are talking about a specific DNA sequence. What this means for you is that you may get a flu vaccine made from a specific strain of the flu virus—let's call this virus A. But the flu that happens to be going around this season is made up of a different virus strain—virus B. If you get a flu shot to protect you from virus A, you are not protected from getting virus B. This basically means that getting the flu shot is kind of a crap shoot. In fact, it may have been somewhat harmful because once you got the flu shot, it suppressed your immune system making you more susceptible to catching virus B!

So let's keep pulling back the curtain to see what else we can find.

Safety:

Pros

We don't need to conduct extensive research to know that vaccines are providing children with some protection, although limited, from disease. Some may argue that it is not as significant as we think but the fact remains that they work. Vaccines are also good at helping to calm people's fears and give them peace of mind. It's a quick fix for the mind. There is an endless and easily accessible body of research on the safety of vaccines. The CDC has several links to recent research addressing the safety of vaccines and the questionable link to autism which can be found at:
www.cdc.gov/vaccinesafety/pdf/cdcstudiesonvaccinesandautism.pdf.

Cons

Anyone who tells you that vaccines are 100 percent safe are dishonest or misinformed. When I hear somebody, whether it's the head of the CDC or the surgeon general, make an exclusive, untrue statement that there are no risks or safety concerns associated with vaccines, I quickly dismiss them as "not credible." There's very little absolute certainty in this world and vaccines do not make it on that short list.

Before we go further, I want you to know that I understand how difficult and overwhelming this process can be. Sometimes when we learn the facts or truths that are hidden from us, we feel betrayed. And it sucks! We all want to believe that our doctors and especially our government would provide us with the information we need to make some tough decisions.

But we live in a time when the information we need is way more accessible than it was ten, twenty or fifty years ago. You no longer have to depend on your doctor or the government to keep you informed. Don't waste your time trying to get others to be accountable...instead be accountable for your own education and seek the truth. It's out there!

You may be surprised to learn that both proponents and opponents of vaccinations agree on this next bombshell of truth about vaccine safety.

What most people don't realize is that the issue of vaccine safety isn't just about what's in the vaccine. That's what everyone likes to argue about because there's so much contradictory research out there. You rarely hear people argue about the serious safety risk of vaccinating a child or an adult with a pre-existing condition.

Why Some People Get Sick After They Get Vaccinated

Imagine your immune system as troop of soldiers. Their main duty and purpose is to fight off any germ, bacteria, virus, or foreign invader that tries to attack the body. They are specialized and highly trained at what they do.

Let's say that your soldiers were busy fighting off an infection and that in order to defeat it, every soldier needed to be engaged in battle. These soldiers were doing such a good job that you didn't really feel any symptoms of infection except for being a little bit more tired than usual.

At this same time, you decide to get a flu shot because you heard on the news that the flu was expected to kill thousands of people this season. Now your soldiers are facing a new foreign invader but don't have enough troops to adequately fight both battles at the same time. So this new virus that you've injected in your body is allowed to explore and spread with no soldiers to stop it. Soon you start to have inflammation, vomiting, or a fever which is the body's natural response to expel toxins and invaders. You are having a reaction that is the direct result of having received a vaccination.

This issue is rarely discussed despite the fact that your child is far more likely to experience adverse reactions to a vaccine due to having a pre-existing condition. There's a warning in every insert of every vaccination on the market today. Government websites dedicate whole pages identifying "people who should not get vaccines." Yet doctors rarely take the time to educate parents about this well-known issue of safety.

If you take away one morsel of information from this chapter, let it be this: You and your child are at a greater risk of experiencing an adverse reaction to a vaccine if you have a pre-existing condition.

Now there are a whole slew of symptoms and conditions known to be adverse reactions and they include:

The mild:
- Fever
- Headaches
- Rash/Swelling at Injection Site

The more serious:
- Allergic Reaction
- Seizures
- Brain damage
- Injury or death

What's more important to know is what is considered a "pre-existing condition." This includes any condition, illness, or use of medication that is/has weakened the body's immune system. For example, if your child has the flu, or is taking a steroidal medication, or you are currently pregnant: all of these conditions would cause your immune system to be weakened or suppressed. So if you or your child were to get a vaccination in this weakened state, it could overwhelm your immune system and result in an adverse reaction.

Here's the problem: we don't always know when our immune systems are compromised. Some children are born with a genetic pre-disposition to an immune disorder or have an under-developed immune system. A pediatrician may be totally unaware there's even a problem because there are no outward signs or symptoms. This is why some children may have an adverse reaction while others don't.

Unfortunately, some doctor's miss the red flags like in the case of my friend. Too often, doctors are busy bouncing from one patient to the next so it's easy to see how such an oversight can occur.

As a social worker, I was trained to identify risk factors that can become barriers to an individual's health and wellness. But I can't predict risk. And neither can doctors and scientists. When a scientist creates a new vaccine or a doctor gives a vaccine injection, they do not have a complete understanding of the unique risk factors for the individual receiving the shot. They don't know the person's pre-disposition, tolerance for chemicals, or their current level of toxicity.

When a pediatrician gives a child a vaccine, rarely do they consider that child's toxic load (the accumulated amount of toxins in the body). They have no way of knowing how the chemicals in the vaccine will contribute to that child's toxic load. Unfortunately, vaccine makers have not invested the time or money to research the impact that vaccines have on a child's already overloaded immune system.

Where I Stand

It may feel like my lists were a little heavy-handed with the cons. And you'd be right for feeling that way. Not because I'm trying to sway you but because my whole purpose with this book is to shed light on the dark matter...meaning the stuff you won't hear on the news. You've already got the government, and doctors, and researchers touting the wonders of vaccines. It's my job to make sure that your information and facts are balanced so you have more control in the decision-making process.

[85]

I went through the same process when it came to deciding what my personal and professional opinions were about vaccines. My decisions are based on what I've learned in school about the human body, our immune system and how it works, the role that diet and nutrition play in our health, as well as a child's developmental needs. It also includes what I have learned from my 20 plus years of experience working with families and medical professionals—plus input from my very good friend who has been a pharmaceutical representative for 20 years (and has asked not to be named for obvious reasons).

I am neither pro-vaccine or what has become known as an anti-vaxxer. I think that some vaccines offer the benefits of prevention yet I believe that the current vaccine schedule is unnecessary and unsafe. I don't think it makes sense to subject a child and their fragile immune system to the onslaught of toxic chemicals. Mind you, chemicals are added to preserve and keep the virus alive and give vaccines a shelf life. These chemicals are not for the benefit of our health.

I believe the most logical approach would be to allow a child's immune system time to develop. At age one, children should be assessed to determine their toxic load (which can be done with a very simple lab test) and for symptoms of any pre-existing conditions. Only then should they be vaccinated.

Children with suppressed immune systems should not be vaccinated but should be prescribed a natural immune boosting diet for a period of no less than six months. Then they can be re-evaluated. It doesn't mean your child will have to live in a bubble. In fact, it will give their immune system the opportunity to develop natural immunity and resistance to bacteria.

I also strongly support and advocate for a parent's right to choose. I am vehemently against giving up that right. I think vaccines are a dangerous form of blind submission. Whenever you surrender your rights, you are essentially giving up control. It doesn't matter if we are talking about vaccines, speech, privacy, or the right to protect your property. Every time you give the government control over one aspect of your life, it is an invitation to erode your individual liberties. The government has practiced this tactic for years. In fact, they are so good at it most people don't even realize when it's happening.

I know I may have lost some of you at this point and that's expected. You may feel an urge to label me as a liberal or a conspiracy theorist. But I promise, I'm not going to ask you to start burning flags or prepping for Hunger Games. What I am trying to do is shatter this idea that we all must believe in the same thing. So often, we have a disagreement with someone and then assume that everything else that comes out of their mouth is nonsense as well. We decide that we can't learn from them if we don't agree with everything they say. I'm

[86]

asking you to be smarter than that; to allow your old beliefs to be challenged for the purpose of becoming empowered.

I don't question the science behind vaccines. I question the practices. I think vaccines are one of the more important medical inventions in history. I do believe that vaccines were instrumental in helping to stop the spread of disease during a time when people were highly susceptible, but today's social climate is very different and the pharmaceutical industry has become tainted by corruption, greed, and profits.

How do you put your trust into an industry where data is manipulated, dissenters are threatened, whistleblowers are silenced, politicians are paid off, and people are injured?

Did you know that if your child is injured by a vaccine that you can't directly sue the maker of the vaccine? You have to go through vaccine court, or, the Office of Special Masters of the US Court of Federal Claims a specialized court that is run by the government. Even if you can prove and win your case, the pharmaceutical company doesn't have to pay.

Financial judgments actually come from government funds which are ultimately funded by us taxpayers. Am I the only one who thinks it's insane that pharmaceutical companies are absolved of any responsibility for their vaccines? No other industry has this kind of immunity…excuse the pun.

As a parent, you are required to take measures to keep your children safe. If you fail to do so, you are subject to being investigated by Child Protective Services and potentially have your child removed from your care. So what if you think a vaccine poses a risk to your child? Don't you have the right and responsibility to protect them? The laws tell you that you do—except when it comes to vaccines. You don't get a say. You've got to rely on your doctor's infinite wisdom and ability to see an unforeseeable health condition that could put your child at increased risk. In the case where children have reactions, seizures, or serious injuries from vaccines, do you think the physician that gave the shots saw any indicators that their patient was at risk? Perhaps, but I doubt it.

I also empathize with doctors because they are under intense pressure to vaccinate. Failing to do so could jeopardize their practice and their reputation. Remember, these professionals have committed a lot of time and money to become doctors. They have too much to lose. I think it must be somewhat disheartening to get into your profession and see it for what it really is. I can relate. I became so disillusioned by the reality of my work that I left.

Like social work, people get into medicine to help other people; not to be dealing with billing codes, government bureaucracy, and non-medical professional like insurance companies and pharmaceutical representatives telling you how to treat people. That's why it doesn't surprise me that some doctors decide that it's easier to go along with the program than it is to fight it.

Being Empowered When It Comes to Vaccines

For starters, be respectful of other parents' decisions: whether it's to vaccinate, delay vaccination, or not vaccinate. Don't expect others to share your beliefs but do expect them to respect it. Recognize that when you mock, ridicule, or pressure others that it comes from a place of fear and uncertainty. Big pharma and its investors (including the government) have purposely planted those fears in your minds for a "peer pressure" effect.

Don't believe me? Then answer this question...if your child is vaccinated against whooping cough and sits in a classroom next to another student who is not vaccinated and has whooping cough, how does the unvaccinated student pose a risk to your child?

The answer is they don't. Unvaccinated children only pose a risk to other unvaccinated children. But here's the kicker! It's possible that your child could get vaccinated for chicken pox and pass the virus on to an unvaccinated child, because the virus can "shed" after vaccination, a recently vaccinated child can pass the virus to a child who has not been vaccinated. But you don't hear about that on the news.

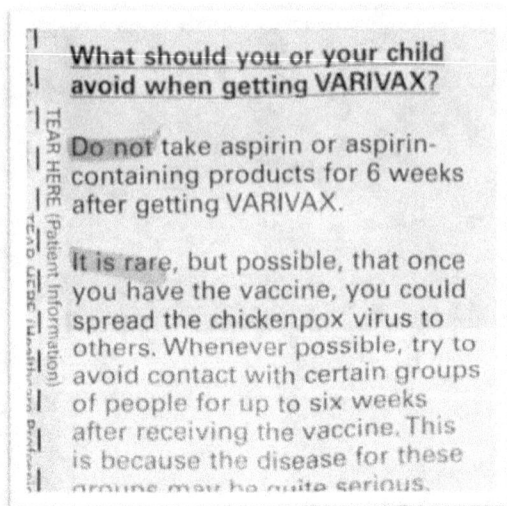

What should you or your child avoid when getting VARIVAX?

Do not take aspirin or aspirin-containing products for 6 weeks after getting VARIVAX.

It is rare, but possible, that once you have the vaccine, you could spread the chickenpox virus to others. Whenever possible, try to avoid contact with certain groups of people for up to six weeks after receiving the vaccine. This is because the disease for these groups may be quite serious.

TEAR HERE (Patient Information)

*A photo of an actual VARIVAX insert for a chicken pox vaccine

I think the most devastating outcome of this debate is how it pits parents against one another. Every parent has the same goal in mind; to raise a healthy child. Raising a healthy child does not require that we all have to agree on how to go about it, but pointing fingers, name-calling, making threats and lashing out in anger does not serve us. It diminishes our power.

"People seem to get violently emotional about vaccinations with a blind, hysterical zeal... Parents bear the responsibility of looking at evidence on both sides. And the most effective way to flush out the truth is to look at the source, the references, and the money(funding). The latter being the strongest indicator of bias. Once educated, I believe it is a parent's intrinsic right to determine if, when, and how they will vaccinate their child."

~ Dr. Tim O'Shea, Author of *The Sanctity of Human Blood*

Know Your Rights

Laws and vaccine mandates vary by state so it's important that you review the current legislation for the state that you live in. Listed below are brief definitions to help you understand exemptions and your right to informed consent.

[90]

Exemptions

Exemptions are granted based on religious, medical, and/or philosophical beliefs. Each state differs on what types of exemptions they allow and the criteria required for qualifying for an exemption.

Informed Consent

You have a right to know what is in the vaccine that is given to your child. Many physicians don't even know this information so you can't always rely on your doctor to educate you. Ask for the vaccine insert. Tell your doctor you want sufficient time to research the ingredients before consenting to your child being injected. Your doctor has the responsibility to provide you with sufficient information in order for you to make an informed choice. This is also a great way to tell how much your doctor really knows and if they support your right to choose. Remember, most physician learn about vaccines from pharmaceutical reps who are NOT trained medical professionals.

Ask Questions

I know it feels uncomfortable and scary to ask your doctor questions but it's a good way to find out just how knowledgeable your doctor is. They will most likely rattle off some general research findings proving that vaccines are safe. Tell your doctor that you are not refusing the vaccinations but need additional information before you proceed. Then ask your physician the following questions:

1. If they regurgitated information from a study, ask for the name of the study, the name of the researcher(s), and if they know who funded the research. Chances are they won't know any of this information. If your doctor gets upset or tells you they don't have time for your questions, you should definitely consider finding a new doctor.

2. Can you have the vaccine insert or a copy of the vaccine insert? It is quite rare that doctors hand these out so don't be surprised if they refuse or say they don't have one. The insert is filled with a lot of technical stuff and fine print that pharmaceutical companies are required to include in packaging but hope you never see. They also encourage doctors not to show the insert to patients as it may confuse us or initiate unwanted questions. Which is precisely why you should ask for it. It will help you to feel empowered and hold your doctor accountable for providing you with information that you are legally entitled to.

3. Do you know how many people in the United States were compensated last year for adverse reactions to this particular vaccination in the past year? The point is to see if your doctor is willing to acknowledge that vaccines do injury some people. Is he or she willing to have a discussion about adverse reactions? They may ballpark it and use terms like "a few," "reactions are rare," "or there's no evidence to suggest." None of these are good responses. A doctor who says, "I'm not sure. I know there are people who are injured from vaccines but I have never had a patient who has suffered such injuries," is a good doctor. I'm looking for that doctor who gives me an actual number or who carefully reviews my child's chart to see if there is any indicator that my child could be at risk. That's the kind of doctor that an empowered parent is willing to give consent too.

The responsibility to be informed doesn't belong solely to your doctor. Here are some important questions you need to answer before making your choice.

What You Can Do to Protect Your Child and Your Rights

- Vaccines can be a shot in the dark. Your child's immune system could be suppressed without your child showing any physical symptoms like a fever or phlegm. If you suspect that your child's immune system is in a weakened state (e.g., history of chronic illness, allergies, unidentified rashes, low energy levels, injuries that are slow to heal) but your doctor insist the child be vaccinated, you can and should seek a second opinion.

- You should never be pressured into giving your child a vaccination. Any doctor who uses fear, intimidation, or makes you feel like a bad parent is not someone you want in your support network. There are plenty of physicians out there who are experienced and support a parent's right to choose.

- If you notice any signs of health deterioration or a delay or regression of development in your child after receiving an injection, it is critical that you report this information to the physician who administered the vaccine. Your child should be closely monitored for any adverse reactions. Document everything and request a copy of your child's medical record. Visit the National Vaccine Information Center at http://www.nvic.org/ to learn more about your rights and what you should do if you believe your hild has been harmed by the injection.

[92]

- You can request a vaccine titer from your pediatrician or an independent lab. A vaccine titer test identifies and measures the antibodies in blood after vaccination or after exposure to the disease by infection. It can tell if your child's level of antibodies are at a "protective" level which means your child has sufficient immunity. Vaccine titers can be used to help you and your physician determine if your child needs additional vaccines. You can order titer test online at Directlabs.com and Accesalabs.com/titer-test.

- If you make the choice to have your child vaccinated, be certain to keep record of which injections your child received, as well as the date and time. Obtain the manufacturer's information and the vaccine lot number. Closely monitor your child for any adverse reactions like the signs and indicators mentioned in the "Safety Pro & Con" section of this chapter.

The more educated you become about vaccines, the more empowered you will become. I know I've thrown a shitload of information your way and hope that you don't feel too overwhelmed. The blunt truth is that I'm not too concerned about which way you decide to go. Ultimately, I just want you to feel confident in your choice. Your decision should be based on the unique needs of your family, not on your fear. We've come a long way from the days of smallpox pandemics. The mumps are not going to wipe out the human population. Drug toxicity perhaps…but not the mumps.

CH. 6 – IN SICKNESS AND IN WEALTH

I used to believe that doctors knew everything. They were the authority on health and it wasn't up to me to question their knowledge. After all, they spent years studying and took out enormous student loans; all to pursue their dream of healing the sick and saving lives. I didn't mind paying for insurance because I liked knowing I had quality healthcare waiting for me should I ever need it. Then something happened.

I eat really healthy so it was difficult for me to understand how, at the age of 31, I found myself dressed only in my underwear, haphazardly covered with a hospital gown, undergoing an electrocardiogram (EKG). I'd driven myself to the ER after convincing my client not to call for an ambulance. It happened while I was lecturing her on abusing her prescription medications. A series of intense chest pains had made me drop to my knees and sent her into a panic. They came and went like contractions, but I had to leave. I preferred the risk of crashing my car to being found unresponsive, covered in cat hair, on my client's dirty floor.

During that drive, I questioned everything about my lifestyle. What was I doing wrong? I'd been healthy and athletic as a young adult and was in great shape for a woman in her early thirties. I was working out more than ever and had just completed a month on the South Beach Diet (the first and last diet I've ever tried). Sure, work had been incredibly stressful but that was the norm. I didn't drink soda and cooked most of my meals, aside from the occasional late Friday night drive-thru chicken sandwich. In comparison to most, I was a longshot for having a heart attack.

By the time I got to the hospital, the pain was so bad that I could barely talk and breathing had become difficult. I will say this, walking into the ER dripping in sweat and clutching your chest is a sure fire way to bypass the waiting room. They took me in immediately and prepared me for the EKG. When the nurse went to place the adhesive discs on my chest, I yelped out in pain. My entire ribcage felt like it was on fire! Every time she touched me it sent ripples of burning pains through my chest.

The doctor was unempathetic and I remember feeling like he lost interest in my condition once he determined it wasn't a heart attack. After the pain medication kicked in, the doctor asked me if I had any other symptoms. I told him about the re-occurring rashes that would appear on my legs and arms that burned and often left scars. There were also the pains I would get in my joints that I just attributed to aging or over-doing it at the gym. And then there were the digestive problems. As if lying on the hospital bed with all my goods on display wasn't embarrassing enough, I told the doctor how things weren't running so smoothly. I mentioned the chronic constipation and the severe cramping that I would sometimes experience in the middle of the night.

Some three hours, later he diagnosed me with *costochondritis,* or in layman's terms, inflammation of the chest wall. Basically the muscles in my chest were inflamed and they were constricting my lungs, which is why I felt the tightness. When I had asked what caused it, he told me that most often it's stress or anxiety. He never really explained the how or why, and he most certainly did not give me any helpful tips on resolving the problem. What he did give me was a prescription for steroids and an anti-inflammatory.

Well, things went straight to Hell from there. I took the steroids which caused me to develop insomnia and made me gain weight. I took the anti-inflammatory which worsened my digestive issues. The lack of sleep made me irritable and depressed. I was miserable. I sought a second opinion from two different doctors, including my primary care physician. One told me I would need to get regular cortisol shots for the pain and the other told me I had major depression and suggested I take an anti-depressant. Neither of these options felt right, so I decided to go with a cheaper and less effective third option. I ignored it and hoped it would go away on its own.

Over the next two years, my health declined significantly. I continued to work but decided to keep a journal of my symptoms. I went from seeing a doctor once a year for my annual check-up to a visit every other month. The frequency of my pain increased as did my rashes. I was diagnosed with anemia, migraines, fibromyalgia, and irritable bowel syndrome for which I was offered a new prescription each time. My life carried on this way until I finally decided to take back control.

I started to read every book I could find on health and nutrition. I read online forums and went to any and every health conference I could afford to attend. That's how I learned about the practice of naturopathic medicine. Naturopathic medicine looks to treat patients by restoring overall health instead of suppressing a few key symptoms with medication. Doctors who practice naturopathy seek to find the underlying causes of symptoms and develop treatment plans that utilize the body's own natural healing mechanisms.

What Is Holistic Health?

Holistic health is the practice whereby a practitioner uses treatments that address the entire body: a person's mind, body, and spiritual needs. It does this by taking an in-depth look at the factors that influence our wellness such as diet, lifestyle, environment, exercise, relationships, and mental health.

I found myself a naturopathic physician. Her name is Dr. Koren Barrett and I hope she doesn't mind that I'm putting her on blast, but she deserves the recognition. Since she wasn't covered by my insurance, I had to pay out-of-pocket for her services. And to this day, it is the best investment I have ever made. She helped me to forever change the health of my body, but more importantly; she showed me what real healthcare should look like. My first appointment with her was for an entire hour. She took copious notes on everything I said and even made copies of pages from my journal to keep on record. She ordered some very simple lab tests to help her figure out what my body was trying to tell me.

Two-and-half years after my visit to the emergency room, I finally got an accurate diagnosis for my condition: toxicity. To put it bluntly, I was full of a bunch of yeast, toxic chemicals, and crap. I was floored, but what was more astonishing was her explanation as to how I became toxic. One of the tests revealed that I had a food sensitivity for all kinds of nuts, especially peanuts. It largely went unnoticed because my reaction was mainly happening internally. See my body, for whatever reason, has a difficult time processing the amino acid arginine, which is found in high concentrations in nuts. This made perfect sense to me since I have had a serious allergy to chocolate my entire life and chocolate is also very high in arginine.

Now, do you remember when I told you that I started having symptoms about one month after I had been on the South Beach Diet? Well, while I was on that diet, I consumed peanut butter on a daily basis. Here I was thinking I was being healthy while in reality, I was making myself very sick. This is not to criticize the South Beach Diet but to point out how important it is that you become proactive in getting to know your body.

There were several other factors that were causing my toxicity, which is basically the process of self-poisoning caused by bacteria, waste, and other poisons being produced within the body.

✓ *Because of my high-stress job, I had chronically high levels of the stress hormone cortisol in my blood.*

✓ *I was dehydrated.*

✓ *I had Candida, an overgrowth of yeast in my digestive tract and as a result, my colon was struggling to absorb nutrients from my food and eliminate waste.*

✓ *I was deficient in vitamins A, D, E, and all the Bs.*

With Dr. Barrett's help, I was able to make a gradual yet radical change in my diet and lifestyle. Four months after that first visit, I was symptom free. I learned that the best healthcare is self-care. Instead of paying for the treatment of my symptoms, I invested time and effort into preventing illness and maintaining health. I still catch a cold once every blue moon, but my body has learned how to heal itself and so I require no medical intervention. I sleep like a baby and weigh the same from year to year. The greatest outcome from that whole experience is my ability to spot poor quality, subpar healthcare like a veteran detective. I chose not to settle, and it changed my life. Now I'm determined to make sure you and your family get the healthcare that you deserve.

Our Current State of Health

Here are some statistics that illustrate the state of health in our country:

➢ Although America is one of the wealthiest nations, we have one of the worst (ranked 46 out of 48) and most expensive health care systems in the world (Mahon, 2014).

[98]

> Over one-third of adults and 17% of youth are obese (Ogden, MD, Kit and Flegal, 2014). There are more obese adults in the US than any other country in the world. (Ng, 2013).

> Over 29 million Americans have diabetes, and of that number, 8.1 million are undiagnosed (American Diabetes Association, 2014).

> Treating Americans for chronic disease such as heart disease, diabetes, and hypertension, accounts for 86 percent of our nation's health care cost (CDC, 2016).

> One in eight children have some form of an emotional or behavioral disorder, with ADHD being the most prevalent (SAMHSA).

> Approximately 38 percent of youth ages 12–17 were diagnosed with a major depressive episode in the year 2013 (Federal Interagency Forum, 2015).

> Medication prescriptions have increased significantly for mental health conditions with the greatest growth for antidepressants for adults and stimulants for children (SAMHSA).

> The 2012 Monitoring the Future study found that 12 percent of high school seniors and 10 percent of sophomores reported having used Adderall, Ritalin, or another stimulant or amphetamine without a prescription at least once (Institute Social Research, 2013).

To sum it up—we are as unhealthy as our healthcare system is inept. We do not live in a society that is conducive to health. Almost everything we do seems to be counterproductive to living a healthy lifestyle. Do you sit at your desk all day staring at a monitor, trapped inside a building that blocks out the sun and fresh air? Do you stay home with young children but find yourself glued to a screen in order to earn income or maintain your social life? Maybe you work outside near a commercial area or roadway where you inhale exhaust fumes all day. We eat on the move or at our desk. We drink caffeinated beverages and sugary drinks to boost our energy because God knows we are no longer energized by the work we do.

You can get more education, you can make more money, you can fall in love over and over again, and you can even create a new life for yourself. But you will never ever get another body.

We didn't just become an adult and fall into this lifestyle. We were trained as kids. Think about it. Schools were great preparation for the work place. Sit at a desk indoors, work, eat fast, get tired, eat sugar to make it through the day, and then repeat for four more consecutive days. No wonder kids have trouble learning and adults are escaping to the internet on their lunch breaks!

We've also been programmed to believe that suffering from chronic health problems is normal, that sickness is a routine part of life that comes with the territory of living. As a nation, we have come to accept disease and illness in our lives like the hideous mole on our back that never seems to go away. We adjust. For example: I want you to think about some ongoing health problem you've had over the years. Maybe it's heartburn, constipation, migraines, or maybe it's gout. You've seen doctors, taken medication for it, been relieved when it went away, and was not at all surprised when it came back. Did you ever really believe you could cure yourself entirely and never suffer another migraine again? Or did you come to accept the condition as a part of your life? I will tell you that the average response is acceptance.

What makes the pursuit and maintenance of health even more difficult is the healthcare system we have in place. Our system is not designed to achieve health. Its primary focus is to profit off the diagnosis and treatment of illness and disease. Even the recent incorporation of preventative care as

Seeking Relief

"Ninety percent of the sore throats we Americans experience each year are viral in nature and immune to antibiotics, but data shows that of the millions that see a physician for a sore throat, nearly two-thirds of patients got a prescription for antibiotics.

Physicians claim that they are only responding to the demands of consumers. But I suggest that it is highly unethical to prescribe a drug that is known for causing adverse drug reactions and for killing beneficial bacteria in the gut, when the patient doesn't even need it." Especially to children who are most at risk of harm.

~ Randall Fitzgerald
The Hundred Year Lie

[100]

a covered service is a weakly-veiled attempt at appearing to be socially responsible.

Insurance companies and health care providers know that most people are reactionary, meaning we react to pain, discomfort, and fear. We are far more likely to take action when we are motivated by one or all of these emotional triggers. When was the last time you reacted to feeling good? Yeah, I thought so. When we are symptom free, we typically don't stop and say to ourselves, "How can I ensure that I sustain this healthy feeling?" The industry knows that there is far more money to be made by reacting to disease than preventing disease.

Our dependence has also steadily increased over the years, thanks to the brainwashing tactics of conventional medicine and the pharmaceutical industry. It's easy to convince people that "there's a pill for that," because the fact is that medicine can save lives. I said it before and I'll say it again, medicine is truly one of man's greatest accomplishments. But too much of a good thing is not only harmful; in the case of medicine, it has the potential to be deadly. The problem is that medical and pharmaceutical industries have managed to convince us that we need drugs to function from day to day. We are constantly being told that we are broken and that only a particular drug can fix us.

How Empowered Parents Manage Healthcare

Know that You Have Options

You can manage your family's healthcare in one of two ways: 1) You can choose the path of least resistance and continue to accept what you are given which includes flu shots that don't prevent the flu, treatments that don't cure, and doctors who only know how to treat with drugs; or 2) You can decide to become proactive and appoint yourself as the team leader of your health network. This second option requires some work on your part but it gives you more control over the outcomes, cost, and team members. Don't worry: there's no right or wrong decision. It really comes down to you deciding what's best for you and your family.

The following are strategies and tools that will help you to feel confident and empowered no matter what you decide.

Create Your Own Healthcare Support Network

What this essentially means is that you are going to do a little mixing and matching. Instead of being stuck with whichever doctor you can, you are going to be very intentional and thoughtful in selecting the professionals who help

[103]

you. It also means that you're open to seeking advice and services from the wellness industry or alternative health care practitioners.

You already know that I seek medical advice from a naturopathic physician, but I also see a doctor through my insurance carrier. Basically, I go to my primary care physician for all covered services like preventative care, yearly exams, wellness check-ups, and any necessary lab work. When it comes to issues of nutrition and treatment, I see my naturopath.

For example, say you take your daughter to her pediatrician for chronic ear infections. The pediatrician runs some tests, gives you a diagnosis, and recommends antibiotics and the possibility of a future surgery. Instead of getting caught up in the vicious cycle of giving your child antibiotics, spend the extra money to see a naturopath or a certified holistic health nutritionist. Instead of treating the symptoms, they can do a more thorough assessment and discover the underlying cause, which often tends to be rooted in diet. Trust me, the small $100-$150 investment you make in that initial visit is worth not having to watch your child suffer or endure an unnecessary surgery.

Do Your Research

Any time you are looking for a new healthcare practitioner, you must qualify them, meaning you must decide if their skills and knowledge meet your unique needs. Research your doctor before your first appointment. There are a number of websites that will help you to investigate your physician's conduct, license status, and experience. The Federation of State Medical Boards has two websites just for that purpose: www.fsmb.org and www.Docinfo.org.

Research the hospitals in your area. Some really horrific stuff can go down in a hospital. Lawsuits, malicious acts by hospital staff, unsanitary conditions, and outlandish charges for routine items and procedures to name a few. If you know ahead of time that you or your child require a hospital stay, take the time to research the facility. If you've got the time to research hotels for that trip to Orlando, then you can find time to research your hospital. Here are a few resources that may help you:

www.Medicare.gov/hospitalcompare/About/What-Is-HOS.html

www.Whynotthebest.org

www.Hospitalsafetyscore.org

Alternative Medicine Options

- **Chiropractic care** – works to restore proper alignment of the vertebrae and spinal cord to assist the body in healing.

- **Environmental medicine** – based on the belief that the causes of illness are found in an individual's surroundings to include food, allergens, (think mold and pollen), and chemicals. These doctors work to identify potential triggers and assist the body in releasing toxins.

- **Herbalist** – An herbalist is a practitioner who uses herbs for medicinal purposes. Herbs have been used for thousands of years in many different medicinal systems and cultures throughout the world.

- **Holistic dentistry** – Holistic dentists take an interdisciplinary approach by using both conventional and holistic treatments to promote dental health. They avoid the use of chemicals and toxins like fluoride and mercury filings.

- **Homeopathy** – Practitioners of homeopathy treat illness and disease on the principle of similarity, which means they believe that small doses of a substance can heal the symptoms caused by a larger amount of the same substance.

- **Osteopathy** – These physicians use manual diagnosis (yes, their hands) and treatments based on the concept of the body being a network of interconnected systems which need to function as a whole. They are trained to assist the body in releasing physical blockages in order to promote healing.

The ultimate goal is to create a support network of trusted service providers that understand and support your health and wellness goals. If you want to get off of medication, then you need a doctor who supports that goal. If you're against having mercury fillings in your mouth, then you'll need to interview and find a dentist who performs toxin-free dental treatments.

The only way you can determine if a provider will respect your choices and concerns is to interview them. Asking clear open-ended questions is an effective way to get to know a potential service provider. Remember, you want a service provider who will inspire, educate and motivate you, so take note of how they communicate and engage with you. It can make all the difference. Whatever you do, don't settle. Your search may feel frustrating, but you owe

[105]

it to your family to explore your options. I promise you, good doctors are out there.

Ideally, you will find a team that will satisfy the needs of your whole family. A team for a family could consist of a pediatrician, family practice physician, internist, ob/gyn specialist, naturopathic doctor, chiropractor, and physical therapist or sports medicine practitioner. Ideally, a few of the practitioners would have worked with each other previously. For example, some naturopathic doctors refer clients to family practice physicians for certain tests or treatments.

Signs You Need to Find a New Doctor

I know you may feel limited in your choices because of the sad truth that our decision-making is so heavily influenced by the type of insurance we have. Let's be real. The pickings are slim; so much so that I once chose a doctor strictly based on the fact that it was the only name I could pronounce. In a perfect world where logic prevails, we should be able to see each doctor's resume. Call me crazy, but I'd also like to know my physician's track record. I happen to know from experience that doctors are human just like the rest of us. They have addictions, mental health issues, character defects, and poor judgment that can seriously impact their quality of care.

Here are six signs that indicate it may be time to shop around:

1. If there are more pharmaceutical reps in the waiting room than there are patients, you need to quit your doctor like a bad habit. When your doctor is being wined and dined by a drug maker, it can have a major impact on his treatment choices. He may decide to prescribe a medication to boost his numbers, not because it's what's best for you.

2. If you are seeing your doctor for weight loss and he struggles with obesity, that's a sign you need to keep looking. That also goes for doctors who smoke.

3. Cut your doctor loose if he is always trying to upsell you to get tests or expensive treatments you don't need. Who does he think he is—a mechanic?

4. Continue your search if he is overly critical of your beliefs, and I don't mean your belief that it's okay to have a daily cheeseburger. I'm talking about your moral beliefs and your preferences for treatment

options. Having letters M.D. behind his name doesn't entitle a person to be sanctified and judgmental.

5. If you've waited for an hour and the doctor spends less than ten minutes with you AND didn't answer all your questions, you need to move on. You deserve the time and attention of your physician. A busy practice is not always the sign of a good practice.

6. If all the pens, mugs, totes, prescription pads, and candies at the reception window bear a Pfizer logo (or any drug maker logo for that matter), they have gone to the dark side.

Why Wellness Exams Are Important

Most standard health insurance plans offer free annual health exams. They are often referred to as "wellness exams", "annual physicals", "routine exams" or "prevention care". This is a great opportunity to check in with all your body systems to make sure things are running smooth. Know that your body has an amazing ability to heal. It will perform and function like it was intended to do as long as you care for it and give it what it needs.

Preparing for Doctor Appointments

We often fall victim to the idea that illness or disease just happens to us. When we get sick or a loved one becomes ill, we tell ourselves that it's out of our control. We get scared and become dependent on the "experts" around us to tell us what to do. Becoming an active participant in your healthcare can help you to restore a sense of control over your body and mind. When you take ownership of your condition, you simultaneously tell yourself that you have the ability to change your circumstances. "I got myself here and I can get myself where I want to be."

So as the leader of your healthcare team, you are in charge of making sure your other team members, like your doctor, have all the information they need to make smart decisions. That's why it is crucial that you show up to your doctor's visit prepared. The kind of care you receive is heavily dependent on the quality of information you provide.

Be Prepared for Your Visit

Make a list of the following:

- Current health concerns
- Current symptoms (have no shame...be as detailed as possible)
- Note how long symptoms have persisted (Ex. days, weeks)
- What seem to be the triggers (Ex. happens whenever I eat eggs, migraines on days I don't drink coffee)
- How often it happens (Ex. 3 times a day, all day long)
- When do symptoms occur...day or night
- What I've taken (list anything you have taken to combat symptoms)
- Note any changes to routine

Make a copy for your doctor and ask him to make this a permanent part of your record. This will hold your doctor accountable and help establish your medical history. Be concise. This will become a permanent part of your medical record so be thoughtful and detailed.

Note all medications you are on, including vitamins and dosages, all healthcare providers you've seen, and contact info if possible.

If you are sick, bring a friend who can take notes while you talk with the doctor. Alternatively, they can ask questions. If your child is sick, it's also helpful to take a friend who can watch your child or siblings so that you are not distracted.

TAKE-HOME NOTES

You should always leave your visit with some notes, whether you take them yourself or ask that your doctor print notes for you. Your take-home list should include:

What test, why, and importance of results
Medications to start, why, and how long
Potential side effects of medications, drug interactions you should know about What should you do if the condition worsens
When is next appointment

Ways to Empower Your Kids

Watching you manage the family's healthcare with confidence is a great way to empower your children. You can show them how remaining calm and taking the time to research and get organized can help them to make smart choices.

It's also important to teach kids how and why they should invest time and effort in their wellness. Explain how eating nutritious foods and taking vitamins is an effective way to prevent illness. It will help them to strengthen their sense of control. It's a wonderfully powerful message that will help kids to realize they have a say in how they look and feel.

Remember that *showing* will have more of an impact on your child than *telling* them what they need to do. This means you may have to make some changes in your behavior as well.

One of the easiest and most effective ways to practice health prevention is with a nutritious diet. Nutrient-rich foods like vegetables, fruits, and plant proteins can actually help you to ward off illnesses by strengthening your immune system. Bond with your kids over making healthy food choices and get them involved in meal preparations.

I've found this works really well with teens who are athletes and want to excel in their sport. They are quite eager to learn about foods that will improve their endurance and strength. You can also teach them how to use foods to help their body heal, like eating high-quality proteins and essential fatty acids to help repair injured muscles.

When you or your child receives a scary diagnosis, you may initially react with disbelief or intense fear. It's not unusual to try to pray or wish it away. Know that in these initial moments, you are vulnerable and susceptible to making a fear-based decision.

We rush to the computer and obsessively search our condition, which often leaves us feeling more scared and confused. Take some time to let it sink in. Talk about your fears together as a family. This is an excellent way to show children how to cope with challenging life events.

Also keep in mind that your doctor's diagnosis is only one person's opinion and a small amount of knowledge. If you were going to buy a house, would you just look at one house and make your decision? No, you wouldn't. Process the fear so you can move past it to a place of confidence and clarity.

Tools to Empower:

Test Results
Get help interpreting your test results. Visit *www.labtestonline.org*

Med Watch Safety Alerts
Stay informed on current safety issues with drugs, medical devices, and medical procedures. *www.fda.gov/safety/medwatch/default.htm*

Medication Guides
Understand medications and their side effects. A comprehensive list of medications and the serious adverse side effects can be accessed at: *www.fda.gov/Drugs/DrugSafety/ucm085729.htm*

New Pediatric Labeling Information Database
A comprehensive database of drugs that the FDA has approved for use with children can be found at:
www.accessdata.fda.gov/scripts/sda/sdNavigation.cfm?sd=labelingdatabase

Mental Health Medications
A comprehensive list of mental health medications is located at:
www.nimh.nih.gov/health/topics/mental-health-medications/index.shtml

Complete list of Nourished Minds resources
www.NourishedMinds.com

The American Board of Internal Medicine, in collaboration with Consumer Reports, has created a website, *Choose Wisely*. It offers a great tool to help patients and parents identify procedures and treatments that may be unnecessary or pose more risks than benefits. They aim to help patients "choose care that is based on evidence, free of harm, not duplicative of other tests or procedures, and truly necessary."

I've included a list (below) of some of the most commonly overused and high risk treatments that they recommend you should question.For access to the comprehensive list, visit
www.choosingwisely.org/doctor-patient-lists/

Commonly Overused Treatments

Antibiotics for Chronic Ear Infections	Antibiotics do not work for ear infections caused by viruses. They also do not help to reduce pain. Overuse of antibiotics can kill of healthy bacteria and cause drug-resistant bacteria to grow. Both bacterial and viral infections will often resolve on their own. During this time, you can use Motrin or Tylenol to ease the pain and inflammation. You can also purchase effective, all-natural remedies from your local health food store.
Antibiotics for Respiratory Illness	Antibiotics do not work on virus-based illnesses. These generally include colds, flu, bronchitis, or sinus infections. Strep throat is a bacterial infection and can be diagnosed with a throat culture and possibly treated with antibiotics.
Sleep Aids for Kids	As I mentioned before, drugs are clinically tested with adults. Drugs that can alter moods and induce sleep (like Ambien and Benadryl) are especially risky when using with children. That's because it's very difficult to determine appropriate dosing and risk of repeated use.
CT Scans	These scans should be used in cases of concussions, severe head trauma, and skull fractures, but not for minor head bumps. If the doctor has ruled out serious injuries or a concussion, then it is not necessary to have your child get a CT scan. CT scans expose your child to cancer causing radiation.
Pap Test/Pelvic Exam	Typically, teens are too young to develop cervical cancer so a Pap Test to assess for abnormal cells is unnecessary. Pelvic exams may be helpful for sexually active teens who present with symptoms of a sexually transmitted infection (STI).

CH. 7 - UPGRADING YOUR PARENTING SOFTWARE

It's not unusual for people that I've just met to confide in me and ask my advice. I'm told that I'm easy to talk to. Maybe it's because I have a genuine interest in hearing people's stories and connecting with them. I've spent years honing my skills of getting into people's business without appearing that I'm getting into people's business. It feels very natural and at times I don't even realize I'm doing it. It's happened with police officers who have pulled me over (and yes, my advice got me out of a ticket), waiting rooms, parties, and especially networking events. A close friend calls it my "gift." She's been with me on many of these occasions and will usually just find a comfortable seat and wait it out. She knows that I like to comfort people and help them to find solutions, even though it may cut into our "girl time." She doesn't sweat me about it because I've been her pro bono counselor for years.

On one such occasion, I was meeting with a business consultant for some financial advice. A few minutes into the conversation I learned he was married with two kids, and I guesstimated somewhere in his late-thirties. He hadn't expected to be on the receiving end of any personal questions, but obliged me anyhow. He was smart and had quickly realized that I was trying to determine if he was qualified to be giving me advice.

After we vetted each other, he asked me about the type of issues I address in my parenting workshops. I told him that I tend to get the most questions and requests from parents for more information on internet safety and technology. He nodded in agreement and said, "Hmm, yeah…. that's interesting because I'm dealing with that very issue with my fourteen-year-old daughter." *Of course you are*, I laughed to myself. He proceeded to share the following story (what I love about Brett's story is that it so perfectly captures the challenges of trying to raise a kid in a digital world).

Brett and his wife had decided to get their daughter, Breanna, a smartphone. She was involved in a bunch of activities outside of school and they figured a phone would help them to keep track of her whereabouts. Not to mention Breanna had laid on the guilt pretty thick and they didn't want her to be a "social outcast" (his words, not mine).

So they got the phone and all went well for a good six months. Then mom had noticed some additional charges on the family's phone bill. It appeared that their daughter had been putting in some full-time hours with the texting and had downloaded a fee-based app. They confronted her about the phone bill and then she did something that truly surprised them. She lied.

Breanna outright denied downloading the app. She also got very "snotty" when they told her she had to reduce her texting. Brett said this type of behavior was very uncharacteristic of their daughter and described her as a good kid, with great grades, who never gets into trouble. He and his wife decided to purchase a monitoring app to track her texts and app usage. He set it up to send alerts to his own phone so that he would get the proof he needed to prove she had lied.

At this point I fought the urge to remind him that he already had proof and was really struggling with the changes in his daughter's behavior—but I let him continue.

Brett went on to explain that the monitoring app was amazing. He felt bad because he was also getting copies of all of Breanna's text messages. What Brett hadn't realized is that the app had a setting which forwarded *all* of her messages to his phone. He and his wife felt like they were violating her privacy. Then he received a series of disturbing texts. Their good, studious, rule-abiding daughter had started exchanging very suggestive photos of herself with a friend.

With a flushed face, he told me how horrified he had been, but mentioned that he was relieved that she was sending them to a girl and not a guy. He said her friend's photos were way worse. How worse I had asked? Semi-nude he replied. Brett had yet to realize that he had an even bigger problem.

In my very calm and direct social worker voice, I had asked Brett if he was aware that he had semi-nude photos of an underage female on his personal cell phone. What had followed was a very long silence as I watched Brett's facial expressions go from confusion, to recognition, to panic all within thirty seconds. Technically, Brett had received and viewed images that under the law, would be considered child pornography. Not on purpose of course, but the images were indeed on his phone.

So I made my very best attempts to diffuse his panic with some humor about me saving him thousands of dollars in bail money. Thankfully he laughed and we were able to come up with some actionable steps he could take to address his daughter's behavior and keep him out of jail.

The moral of this story is to stress how important it is for you to upgrade your parenting software. You don't have to become a tech guru but you must learn the basics and get educated on how kids are using technology these days. This is especially crucial if you have kids between the ages of eight and seventeen, which is the age group we'll be focusing on for the purpose of discussion.

I know you may be thinking, *I've got too much "real life" stuff to deal with and don't have time to worry about apps, and games, and filters, and*

Giving Up Your Right to PRIVACY

Did you know that every time you download an app on your phone and click to AGREE that you are essentially giving the app access to your phone's content? That means the company that makes the app can look at your contacts, location, and even your text and photos!

They do this to gather more information about you like who your friend's are, where you shop, what you like. The company can then sell this information to other companies who will start placing ads in your searches and on the sites you visit.

Many of these apps will run in the background gathering data when you're not even using your phone.

Do you know which apps your child has downloaded on their phone?

These apps may be free but you and your family are definitely paying a price!

privacy! I get it; it feels like I'm just cramming more stuff into that already heavy backpack of responsibility that you're carrying around. The truth is, you can't afford to think that way anymore. None of us can. Whether you like it or not, technology is and will continue to be an integral part of our daily lives. We've got to learn to manage it in order to stay in control.

Why You Never See Your Kid's Face Anymore

There's nothing inherently different about kids today. They are curious, imaginative, evolving, self-centered, and vulnerable just like us when we were their age. Yet the world we live in has changed dramatically. As a result, children have had to adapt to the new social norms and rules of engagement. Thankfully, children are far more flexible and adaptable than us adults. They embrace change with the excitement of—well, a child. It's their nature.

In today's world; kids learn, communicate, and socialize online. You must also understand that the social development for school-age kids is focused on learning how to relate with the outside world and the people in it as well as to identify who they are in this world. It's heavy stuff.

Kids are trying to self-identify and figure out "who they are." One of the ways they do this is by seeking out connections and friendships with peers. While school campuses continue to be a great place for kids to meet, the digital world extends their reach across the globe. It fulfills their basic human need for connection and acknowledgement in addition to fulfilling their desire for excitement and escape.

These are the very reasons why you MUST set rules and monitor their life online. When something meets our basic needs AND fulfills our desires all at the same time, it becomes a powerful force in our lives. When it gets too powerful, we run the risk of becoming dependent on it and/or addicted to it.

Consider the power that drugs have over an addict's life, or when a person's love for their partner gets so strong that they become powerless to end a bad relationship. We struggle with this as adults, so you can imagine how challenging it is for a kid to not get sucked in. They don't yet have the insight to understand this dynamic. If you're not there to guide them and help them find a healthy balance, they could lose themselves in a world they can't fully understand.

The biggest challenge with kids and technology is that kids aren't really developmentally mature enough to deal with the emotional aspects of advanced technology. Sure they know how to navigate it and use it, but they don't fully understand it. What I mean is that kids often lack the comprehension, judgment, foresight, and emotional competence to live life

[116]

online. This is mainly because so much of the content on TV, in videos, on social media, and even in games is adult in nature.

This shows up in the form of racking up cell phone charges, losing expensive phones, telling strangers private information, sharing intimate photos, bullying, and coercion into unsafe behavior.

Some dismiss such behavior as kids doing stupid stuff. I say it's kids being kids. It's only stupid when we expect kids to act like adults (and mature ones at that).

Protecting Your Child's Privacy

The Children's Online Privacy Protection Act (COPPA) aims to help parents protect their children's privacy. The rule states that websites must notify a parent of kids under the age of thirteen before collecting, using, or disclosing that child's personal information. I don't know how they determined thirteen to be the cutoff, because I know some very immature sixteen-year-olds, but it's a start. The government is trying to keep up with technology which is not so easy. The Federal Trade Commission enforces this law so be sure to contact them if you think a website is in violation.

*If you need to file a privacy complaint visit: Ftc.gov/complaint

The online world can also give kids (and adults) a false sense of anonymity, like they are saying and doing things behind an invisible wall of protection. It's what allows people to detach themselves from their behavior. It's also what makes it difficult for kids to hold themselves accountable.

How Empowered Parents Manage Technology

Here are some strategies for protecting your kids online:

- Talk with your child and start early. If you think they're old enough to be online, then they're old enough to have the discussion. Don't wait for them to initiate. Use stories from the news or your community to get the conversation going.

- Set rules and expectations. Setting clear boundaries should give your child examples of acceptable and unacceptable behavior, while giving appropriate consequences will help you to manage and modify their behavior. Involve them by asking them to create realistic rules. This will encourage accountability and make the process more democratic.

- Periodically review their text and instant messaging. Make it a habit to regularly review their computer history to see which destinations they are visiting. Explain that this is not about trust vs. mistrust, but that it is the best way for you to determine that they are acting responsible and respectful of your rules.

- Ask them if they know every single one of their Facebook friends. This is especially important for younger teens. Explain the risk of "friending" people they don't know.

- Keep the desktop computer in a common area of the home so that you are better able to monitor usage.

- Set times of restricted use. For example, all cellphone and digital electronics go in your room or office on the charger by 10 p.m. every night.

- Use parental controls. Remember, it is your responsibility to monitor and set limitations. I am giving you my permission to get in their business. Use blocks to block certain websites or special browsers that filter out inappropriate sites. Don't let your child guilt you and most certainly don't listen to other moms who try to make themselves feel better by judging you.

- Be patient. You may already be familiar with what this looks like. It's your parrot impression where you constantly repeat yourself. Kids need to hear things more than once before they get it so have some patience.

- And one of my favorites…listen. It's powerful and amazing what you can learn about your child by doing this. Believe it or not, listening encourages them to actually share more.

Topics to Discuss with Your Teens

Equally important as protecting your child is having the following discussions with them. Someday they will leave the protection of your household, and your conversations, even if not fully understood by them, will set a standard for their behavior. They will also lay the groundwork for your child in terms of speaking to their own children about similar topics someday.

Privacy

Encourage your teen to get a friend's okay before they share a picture or video of them. Getting permission demonstrates that they respect their friend's privacy.

[120]

Accountability

Hammer it into their heads that they relinquish control of a picture once they post it. It doesn't matter if they send it to a friend's phone or post it on social media; it's out of their hands so to speak. Encourage them to only post pics they wouldn't mind being seen by their teacher, coach, college administrator, or future employer.

Explain that online actions have real life consequences. If you wouldn't say it in-person to someone's face or a room full of people—then don't write it online.

Sexting

Teens think it's harmless and parents don't believe that their kids are doing it. Yet sexting or the act of using a phone or digital device to send intimate or sexually explicit text or photos is more common than you think. And it can land your teen in serious trouble with the law.

So what do you get when you cross a curious teen with raging hormones and the alluring anonymity of text messaging? You guessed it; Sexting!

It gives teens the courage and false sense of maturity to say something that they would never otherwise say face-to-face. To them, it is easy, fun and makes them feel grown up. As a parent, you need to know that sexting is risky behavior and can result in both long-term emotional consequences and criminal consequences.

What's Behind the Behavior? The National Campaign to Prevent Teen and Unplanned Pregnancy defines "sexting" as the act of sending or posting provocative or sexually explicit personal images, video or text via a cell phone or other electronic devices.

The National Campaign conducted one of the first studies of its kind and found that sexting mainly occurs among teens ranging in age from 13-19.

Eye-opening findings of the study to consider:

- 20 percent of teens surveyed reported that they have sent/posted nude or semi-nude pictures or video of themselves

- 37 percent of teen girls admitted to sending/posting sexually suggestive messages

- 39 percent of teen boys admitted to sending/posting sexually suggestive messages

[121]

- 66 percent of teen girls and 60 percent of teen boys reported that they did so to be fun or flirtatious

- 25 percent of teen girls and 33 percent of teen boys reported that they have had nude or semi-nude images shared with them despite the fact that these images were originally sent to someone else

- 51 percent of teen girls reported feeling pressure from a guy to send sexy messages or images

As a parent, you need to be aware of the legal ramifications of sexting. *According to the National Conference of State Legislatures, any image or photo containing some form of nudity of a child under the age of 18 can automatically be considered child pornography.*

Many states have already enacted legislation that calls for serious charges to be brought against anyone, regardless of age, who distributes, sends, or takes such images.

Teens often don't have the maturity and forethought to realize that once they put such a picture on the internet it can be accessed and used by anyone. What they thought was an innocent act can lead to harassment, intimidation, public humiliation, or the risk of it falling into the hands of someone with malicious intent. Be sure to talk with your kids about the dangers of cyberspace and social media sites. It's important to know who your teens are communicating with and to clearly express your expectations for appropriate behavior.

Be aware that many phones come with tracking applications that can track the phone's location or attach the location of the user to images that are then shared. The *pro* of this feature is that it can help you to find a lost phone or help you to locate your child. The *con* is that it can also help other people locate you or your child. If this feature has been activated on your child's phone or within an application—let's say Instagram—any photo that your child takes will have the location of the photo embedded in the data of the image. In other words, if your child takes a picture in their bedroom and posts the photo to Instagram, anyone who knows about this feature can do a little research and find out where your child lives.

Most mobile phones also have parental controls. If you've discovered that your child has engaged in reckless phone use, you can turn off apps, texting or downloading features. If you suspect inappropriate behavior, set limitations and restrictions and always remember that having a cell phone is a privilege…not a right!

[122]

Cyber Bullying

Teens spend a tremendous amount of time on their digital devices. This means that a good majority of their social interactions are happening online, which puts them at a greater risk of having an online experience that threatens their emotional well-being. Unfortunately, social media sites like Twitter, Instagram, and Facebook can serve as useful means for people to spread their hateful and hurtful beliefs and messages. Bullying has spread from school campuses to the online world where its potential for harm is magnified. We must recognize that cyberbullying is not simply "kids being kids" but a larger social and cultural issue that has extreme consequences for both the bullies, the bullied, and parents.

There are many different types of behaviors that fall under the umbrella of bullying:

> **Harassment** – The repeated act of sending threatening or offensive messages to a victim to incite fear or humiliation. It may involve a bully finding out personal information about the victims such as email address, phone number, or home address and then using this information to stalk or harass the victim. This can also include outing which is the act of posting or publishing personal or private details about the victim within a social group or network circle.

> **Flaming** – The act of instigating an argument or conflict by taunting the victim with the hopes of getting a response. Typically, this is done through social media so that the bully has an audience and the victim is made to look like a coward or is shamed for not defending themselves.

> **Exclusion** – The act of ignoring, blocking, or freezing the victim out of a social group. The bully often encourages others to cut off contact with the victim which can be intensely traumatizing for most teens.

> **Impersonation (a.k.a. Masquerading)** – The act whereby the bully creates a false profile or identity to post or publish hateful or hurtful messages about the victim. Bullies tend to resort to impersonation after their original profile was blocked or their account was deleted/deactivated by a webmaster. Other times bullies will masquerade as an attempt to remain anonymous.

[123]

The Empowered Way to Deal with Cyberbullies

Don't engage the bully. People who bully other people online (trolls) do so to make themselves feel powerful. It serves as a great distraction from their own unhappiness and is usually an indicator that they feel unaccepted in the real world. It is way easier to cut someone else down than it is to acknowledge your own insecurities.

If your child is being bullied online, the best reaction is no reaction. When you feed into the behavior, you help to make the bully feel powerful. A response actually fuels their behavior because it gives them the very thing they want most…attention. Teach and show your teen how to be empowered by "going dark" on the bully.

If the bullying persists, you can get proactive by documenting, recording, and tracking the bully's behavior so that you can file a report with the authorities. You can also use this information to report to the webmaster of a particular site since they have the power to delete the bully's account. Most websites have a direct email address for this purpose. If not, you can go to the contact page and use the email address. This is an awesome way to help your teen learn how to overcome adversity and develop confidence and coping skills.

If your child is the bully, you need to sit them down and have a heartfelt talk about their motivation. I guarantee you there is always an underlying issue of low self-worth, insecurities, a need to be accepted, or some unresolved pain. People hurt others to mask their own pain.

Tools for Empowerment

CommonSenseParenting.org
This is an awesome website! I highly recommend it to any of you that worry about the content of the movies, games, and apps your kids watch and use. Their movie review system rates movies based on their language, violence, and sexual content, as well as the movies' positive messages and positive role models. It does the same with apps, books, games, and TV shows. This site also has a great section called "Parent Concerns" with research-based FAQs and guidance for parenting in the digital age.

NetFamilyNews.org
A blog to educate and support parents on issues of internet safety and youth-related technology.

ConnectSafely.org
Website dedicated to educating users and parents on issues of internet safety, privacy and security. A great resource with research-based safety tips, parent guidebooks, and advice on all aspects of tech use and policy.

NetSmartz.org
This is one of my favorite sites to refer parents too because it's interactive and makes learning fun. It has educational videos and games for kids to practice online safety and learning. It also has great guides and videos for parent to learn how they can protect their kids and use the internet as an educational tool.

My Mobile Watchdog
Records text messages sent and received from your child's phone that you can print and review or use to confront inappropriate behavior. It's hard to lie when the evidence is in print.

Mobile Spy
Undetectable software you can load onto your child's phone which silently uploads data to your Mobile Spy account. It is a safer alternative to the app I shared in Brett's story. Rather than text coming straight to your phone, it gets stored in an account.

iProtect for iPhones
Monitoring system that logs instant message conversations; you can set it up to run at specific times.

Does Your Kid Need a Smartphone?

Cell phones are a good way to stay in touch with your child when they are out there in that great big world without you. Which brings up the very debatable question: When should you get your child a smartphone of their very own? Now I happen to think that you are the expert on your own child.

There is no one better equipped to determine when you should grant your child this privilege, but make no mistake—having a smart phone is a privilege. Yes, it does make it easier for you to monitor your child's safety and whereabouts, but you can also keep your child safe without one. The only thing they will suffer from is an exaggerated sense of embarrassment and entitlement.

Of course they want a phone because evvvveryone has one, but that alone is not a good enough reason. Keeping up with the Joneses is how you breed entitlement in your child. Not the lesson we're going for here. This decision requires some thoughtful evaluation, especially taking into account your child's level of maturity.

The good news is that you have options. There is always the option of getting your child a basic phone that only makes calls. This way you can have a trial run and give them the opportunity to demonstrate that they are responsible and ready for something with more capabilities.

If you are considering a smart phone, the three biggest factors you want to assess for when making your decision are:

1. Has your child demonstrated responsible use of the internet on your home computer and respected your rules of usage? This is critical because your child will essentially be walking around with a mini computer. You need to be certain that he or she will follow the same rules for privacy, content, and sharing of information/photos.

2. Can you afford it? The simple fact is your child does not **need** a smart phone. These phones are not cheap and as you know, kids don't really understand roaming, app fees, and text overage charges. Not to mention that kids drop and lose things on a daily basis. Really make sure it is in your budget and refrain from doing it out of guilt and pressure.

3. What is YOUR need? This is not about making life easier for them. They have it pretty good already, but getting them a smart phone should be about making it easier for you. If it brings you a sense of peace and security to know that you can reach your child by text, a phone call, receive a photo of them as "proof of life," or note their exact location with GPS, then pull the trigger. All the other apps and features are bonuses and kids should be instructed how to use them wisely.

Remember, age is not really the issue. It's about responsibility, cost, and need. Don't let the moms at soccer practice make you feel bad if you don't think the time is right. This is your call to make.

[126]

App Aptitude

Trying to stay ahead of the techonology game could cause you to go insane. But learning the basics about digital gadgets and software can help you to protect your family's privacy. The best place to start is by getting more familiar with how apps work on smartphones. Careless use of apps can put you and your kids at an enormous risk for privacy violation.

What You Need to Know

- Apps collect data from your phone like contact information and websites you've visited.

- Apps sell this information to other businesses.

- Apps place ads within other apps to get you to buy stuff.

- Apps may charge you money, even if they are free.

- Apps do not always fully disclose what information they collect.

- Apps may store your data on their servers for years and years.

- When you give consent or agree to "terms of use", you essentially give apps the freedom to roam through your phone's data storage looking for useful information to sell.

- Apps can stay on even if you've turned your phone off.

CH. 8 – THE NEW STRANGER DANGER

By far, my most favorite part of my job as a social worker was interviewing kids. Nothing made me happier than those moments when I could make a child smile or laugh, especially when it felt like their world was crumbling around them. As we get older and start lugging more emotional baggage around with us, we tend to lose that connection to our inner child. I find that to be so unfortunate, but I discovered that talking with a child had the magical effect of making me feel child-like again. Even if it was for just a moment.

I know you can relate to what I'm saying because you've had those moments too, like when your child has done or said something crazy and you couldn't even discipline them because you were too busy laughing or trying to get it on video, or in those wonderful moments we allow ourselves to take a trip with them into imaginary worlds where adult problems don't exist.

The reality of my job was that I was usually meeting these children in the midst of a crisis. Many of these families were experiencing the damaging effects of divorce, domestic violence, mental illness, and drug and alcohol abuse. The thing you have to remember is that when you're going through some stuff, your kids are going through it with you. I know it feels better to think that you are shielding them and protecting them but trust me, they know

[129]

something is up. They are far more aware than you realize. They will sense and feel the stress and tension in the house and they will internalize it.

It's actually quite common for some parents to unknowingly project their fears onto their children. That's how kids inherit some of their habits and beliefs. I found that a parent's behavior often has a profound effect on a child's ability to cope. You already know that your children are always watching you. Whether you want to own it or not, you're in a constant state of role modeling how to behave for your child. This is especially crucial when it comes to coping with stress or a crisis. Your kids learn how to cope by watching how you respond to different life events and experiences. This becomes a part of their blueprint.

I was really intrigued by this dynamic because I started to notice that the kids with stronger coping skills seemed to be more aware of potential dangers. For example, I had this standard part of my interview where I assessed a child's ability to cope in a dangerous or unsafe situation. I'd give them several different scenarios and then ask them what they would do in each situation. The scenarios differed based on the child's age but it always included situations of being approached by a stranger, being lost, being touched inappropriately, or witnessing some kind of violence.

Not only was this an effective assessment tool, it also happened to be highly entertaining. I mean, out of the mouths of babes! You wouldn't believe some of the replies I heard.

These are some actual responses I've heard from kids over the years.

One little boy who was about seven-years-old at the time of our interview told me what he would do if an adult stranger (I should note that he asked me to clarify if the stranger was a kid or an adult. He wanted a lot of detail in order to formulate his response which just made me laugh on the inside) try to grab him. First, he would hit him in his nuts. I should note here that he emphasized "real hard." If that didn't work and the "bad guy" pulled him into his car, he would quickly find a penny and shove it into the place where the key goes so the "bad guy" wouldn't be able to start the car. Are you kidding me?! I swear, I'm not making this up. All of his answers were like that. Well, in some of them he possessed superpowers, but for the most part, this kid was prepared for whatever craziness life tried to throw at him.

A cute, curly-haired six-year-old shared her safety plan with me while we threaded bead bracelets in her Disney princess-themed bedroom. With her mother standing directly outside the open bedroom door, I asked the little girl what makes her feel unsafe or scared. She replied that she gets scared when her dad yells and calls her mom bad words. She said she knew they were bad words because they would make her mom cry. I asked her what she does when this happens. She told me that she locks herself in the bathroom or gets into bed and pretends that she's asleep. While we were talking, I could hear her mom softly sobbing in the hallway.

When asked what he would do if he got lost in a store, a five-year-old boy replied that he would go find his mom. When I reminded him that he didn't know where she was in the store, he said that he would ask for help. I then asked what he would do if a man found him and said he knew where his mom was at. He said he would follow the man to get to his mom (you'd be surprised how many kids answer this way!).

A twelve-year-old boy who was home by himself when I made an unannounced home visit actually invited me inside the house to wait for his parents. I told him that it's not safe to have strangers (even female strangers) inside the house when his parents were away. He agreed with me and then proceeded to walk out onto the doorstep and close the front door behind. He actually thought it would be much safer to go outside with a stranger!

I was once involved in an investigation with a thirteen-year-old girl, still in junior high-school, whose parents were concerned that she had been sexually molested. They had found her journal where she kept a running log of all the different sexual acts that she had been engaging in with different boys at school. Her parents were mortified because her entries were so detailed and casual in her accounts. After my interview with the girl, law enforcement decided that no crime had occurred since all those involved were minors of the same age. However, a crime of a different nature had definitely taken place. This confused and naïve young lady admitted to me that she did it for the attention. She had felt isolated and invisible and in order to cope with the lack of attention, she gave the only thing that she thought boys wanted from her. She pretended that she liked doing sexual stuff when she really didn't and figured that even though other girls talked bad about her, at least they knew who she was.

I could go on and on, but I'm hoping you see my point. My interviews essentially became my own personal research project into understanding why some kids seemed aware while others seemed to be at an increased risk of harm.

What was most surprising to me was the discovery that a good majority of kids had no idea what they would do in a crisis or unsafe situation. I got a

[131]

lot of blank stares and "I dunnos" when I asked kids my safety questions. This lack of awareness wasn't just an age thing. I watched teens fumble with their responses or dismiss the possibility that something would ever happen to them. It was alarming and a clear indicator that these very important conversations were not happening at home. I asked the parents of these kids if they were talking to their children about sex, molestation, violence in relationships, drugs and alcohol, bullying, and depression. Can you guess what they told me? Well, if you answered, "No," you'd be right. I really appreciated their honesty—in fact, I thought it was brave. It takes a strong person to acknowledge that they need to grow and improve. Their openness and willingness to learn also helped me to become a better educator and coach.

In fact, the valuable information that you're learning about in this chapter is based on what I learned from those families. You can't get this type of insight from teachers or from sitting on a therapist's couch. What I'm sharing with you comes from nearly fifteen years of interviewing thousands of parents and children. The goal is to save you time, money, heartbreak, and sleepless nights by learning from their mistakes and successes. To do that, we're going to talk about the "where I should put my focus" and the "what can I do" regarding safety and protection.

I could write an entire book on this subject alone, but I think I've scared you enough already. To make good use of our time, let's just focus on the fundamentals. Then I'll give you some practical advice and effective strategies that you can easily incorporate into your parenting repertoire.

The Ten Most Common Responses from Parents When Asked Why They Don't Talk to Their Kids About Safety and Protection

1. It makes me uncomfortable and feels awkward.

2. I don't know if I'll be able to answer their questions.

3. They may tell me something I don't want to know.

4. I don't want to scare them or make them anxious.

5. They don't ever ask me about those things.

6. I'm not sure they're old enough.

7. I wanted to but just never found the time and kept putting it off.

8. They learn about that stuff in school.

9. My kid doesn't listen to me.

10. I'm pretty sure they know more than I do.

Did any of those ring true for you? Listen, I'm on your team so can we be real with each other? All of those reasons are just really great excuses to avoid a potentially uncomfortable conversation. I want you to imagine what it would feel like having to talk with your child after they've been bullied or victimized.

I can tell you that parents struggle with the guilt that comes from wondering if they could have prevented it. I say why wait and do damage repair when you can potentially avoid danger altogether? From now on, that's your goal—prevention.

The first step in prevention is getting over yourself and all of your own fears. You need to put all that baggage aside or in the overhead compartment for a minute and be fully present for your child. It's normal and okay to be nervous or feel unprepared, but don't let that stop you from initiating a discussion.

Your actions are probably even more important than what you say because the way children respond to fear, crisis, challenges, and adversity in life is usually a learned response. If you avoid sensitive topics and let your fear stop you from taking action, you're likely to pass on those behaviors to your child.

How to Be a Positive Role Model

1. How you go about your day-to-day interactions offers the best opportunity to model positive behaviors

2. Make sure your actions are consistent with your words

3. Show respect to others even when angry or frustrated

4. Acknowledge your imperfections, and apologize and admit mistakes

5. Demonstrate healthy ways of coping with adversity and stress like exercise, taking action, coming up with solutions

6. Think out loud so your child can learn how you work through problems, weigh pros and cons, and come to a decision

7. Get outside your comfort zone and be open to trying new things

8. Be confident and proud of who you are.

[133]

However, if you are the type who can move past the fear to do some problem solving and planning, you are likely to encourage those type of coping skills in your child.

Take our seven-year-old with the penny for example. He was a problem-solver who had all kinds of plans of what to do in a crisis. When I met with his parents and told them about their son's response, they laughed. They explained that they think he got the penny idea from a movie but admitted that they are always talking to him about safety and being aware of his surroundings. Mom noted that it helps that he has an older brother who gives him daily lessons on how to beat up "bad guys." His parents were aware of their fears but spent less time worrying and more of their time talking to their kids about scary situations and what they should do when something happened.

Bottom line is this: the way you cope and deal with adversity and crisis has a direct impact on your child's awareness and their ability to problem solve and cope with stressful situations. These also happen to be the very skills your child needs in order to recognize when they are in harm's way and find the courage to take action to protect themselves.

I hate to sound like a Sports Center commentator, but your child's best defense is their offense. As their coach, you don't want to send them into the game unprepared.

So for the remainder of this chapter, we're going to identify the biggest threats to your child's safety and well-being. Then I'm going to teach you what I learned from the extraordinary parents I've met over the years. They took some very simple actions that kept their kids safe and even saved their kids' lives. Lastly, we'll talk about why trying to protect your kids from everything can actually do more harm than good.

When a Stranger Calls

Do you remember the movie, *When a Stranger Calls*? There was a remake of it in 2006 but the original came out in 1979. I feel compelled to take a sidebar and note that I was way too young to watch the movie when it first came out, but I saw it years later when I was seventeen.

I'm not a big fan of blood and gore horror movies but I do love a psychological thriller. You know, the kind of movie that will make a logical grownup sleep with the lights on. The more realistic the better. Which is what I loved about this movie because you could imagine this shit really happening!

I won't give too much away, but it's about this teenage girl who is babysitting when she starts to receive a series of calls from a stranger who tells her she's being watched. Well, in one horrifying climatic moment the girl

[134]

realizes that the calls are coming from inside the house. Oh man, I get anxious just thinking about it!

I make mention of this movie because it reminds me so much of the shift that has occurred when I think about the biggest threats to the safety and well-being of children. The fact is that "stranger danger" is not really the danger you need to be worried about. That's because most of the time when a child is victimized, the perpetrator is usually someone they know.

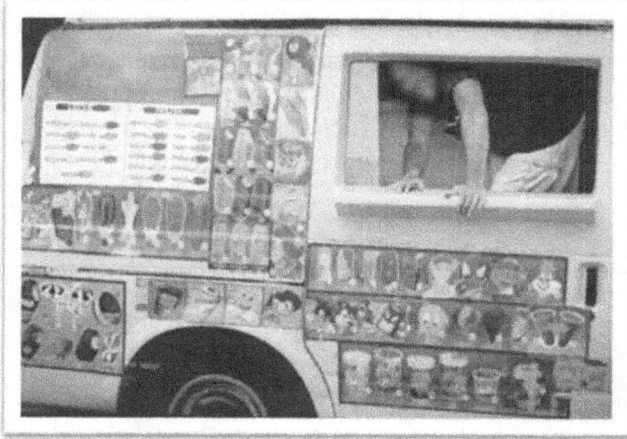

Remember when this guy was all you had to worry about!

The good news is that you don't have to worry so much about the creepy ice cream man. Actually, let me clarify that. You still need to keep your kids away from him. While there is a very small chance that he will abduct your child, there is a significant risk that he will aid and abet in your child's development of obesity or diabetes.

That said, I know that child abductors masquerading as ice cream men is a classic nightmare for parents, but you've got bigger problems to deal with. The scary truth is that the biggest threats to your child's safety and well-being are already inside your home. The stranger is inside your house!

According the report, *National Incidence Studies of Missing, Abducted, Runaway, and Thrownaway Children in America,* complied by the Department of Justice (who comes up with these report titles?!) (Flores, 2002), abduction by strangers is not very common. Even though these findings were published over a decade ago, the numbers continue to remain relatively the same.

➢ Of the majority of cases of missing children, nearly 90 percent are the result of kids getting lost, misunderstanding plans, or running away.

[135]

> Approximately 9 percent are kidnapped by a family member in a custody dispute.
> A very small minority, 3 percent, are abducted by non-family members, but in many cases the child knows or has met the perpetrator before.
> Only about 1 percent of abductions are committed by a stranger and it is estimated that about 50 percent of these children come home.

What this tells us is that it's time to let go of the belief that teaching kids to be wary of strangers is how we protect them. In reality, they are at much greater risk of violence at the hands of a caretaker, or emotional harm from an online bullying, or physical harm from the foods they eat and the cars they drive. For the purpose of putting things into perspective, I need to get a little dark on you.

The following is a list of the top five causes of death for kids under the age of eighteen (not in any special order):

1. Genetic conditions present at birth

2. Accidents (unintentional injuries such as drownings and traffic accidents)

3. Homicide (typically at the hands of a caretaker)

4. Cancer

5. Suicide

You know what all of these things have in common? Each may be somewhat preventable. Certainly, it is worth our best efforts to at least try to prevent them.

We have scientific evidence linking cancer to environmental toxins, chemicals, and poor diet. It is even possible to prevent some genetic conditions with pre-conception healthy diet and lifestyle. Some 390 children die each year from accidental drownings, many of which could have been prevented by simple measures such as requiring life jackets while boating, or installing a self-closing, childproof safety fence around the family pool.

Child abuse can be prevented and stopped with an intervention to address a parent's mental health issues, drug use, or violent tendencies. In most cases, suicide is always preceded by some signs of depression, isolation, or withdrawal. What this tell us is that you as a parent, have the ability to prevent or at least reduce the risk of the five biggest threats to your child's life. You don't need to be a doctor or a social worker. You just need to be aware.

The best way to strengthen your ability to protect your child is to shift your mindset from fear/reaction to one of awareness/prevention. You should be giving yourself a fist bump right now because you're already there. Reading books like this one, in order to get informed, is exactly how you become aware. The prevention piece of the puzzle is where you take action. We already covered some prevention strategies in previous chapters that you can use to prevent health hazards like chronic disease and drug misuse. Now let's explore what empowered parents can do to protect kids against today's increasing threats.

How Empowered Parents Protect Their Kids

Protection Against Sexual Predators

In chapter 7, we discussed what you can do when your child is being bullied at school or online. To make sure that we're covering all bases, we also need to talk about the threat of sexual predators.

Child predators existed long before we had computers, but the internet has made it super easy for them to get access to your kids. It allows them to seek and pursue victims virtually undetected. Perhaps the biggest concern is that they can interact with your child and form a connection or friendship, all while being anonymous or posing as a peer.

I want to make the distinction between sexual predators and pedophiles. People who commit sex crimes against children aren't necessarily pedophiles. Sexual predators do not specifically target prepubescent children, rather they tend to seek out adolescent females and males (less often). Pedophiles tend to have multiple victims and often have a specific preference for prepubescent male victims.

Online sexual predators are looking for specific behavioral traits and emotional vulnerability in a potential victim. This is what allows them to establish an emotional relationship which they use to persuade, entice, or coerce a kid into engaging in sexual acts both on and offline. This manipulation

[139]

technique is also referred to as "grooming." These predators will work very hard to gain a kid's trust and drive a wedge between the kid and their family. Keep in mind, this information is also applicable to sexual predators offline as well.

Behavioral & Emotional Traits that Increase Your Child's Risk of Being Victimized

- Child spends a considerable amount of time online, especially on social media and in chat rooms.

- Child has long periods of unsupervised time alone, whether during the day or at night.

- Child is isolated and has few friends, no friends, or struggles with social awkwardness.

- Child is anxious to have a boyfriend/girlfriend and seeks attention from the opposite sex.

- Child is naïve, gullible, or easily manipulated by others.

- Child has acted out sexually with a peer or adult.

7 Signs Your Child Is Being Victimized (this is not an inclusive list nor a guarantee; they are indicators that warrant further investigation)

1. You find pornography on their computer or phone. It may be adult pornography, which is often used as a way to get your child comfortable talking about sex.

2. Your child receives late night texts, emails, or voicemails from an unfamiliar individual or someone using a moniker, nickname, or who remains unidentified (for example 1-800 numbers, initials only, or uses screen name instead of actual name).

3. Messages are in code or encrypted (meaning you need a password to view the actual text).

4. Your child receives gifts or packages from someone you don't know.

[140]

5. Your child is acting secretive and does suspicious things like turning the computer off quickly, closing the laptop abruptly, hiding the phone, or locking the phone. Your child may stop talking when you enter the room, or talk in code.

6. Your child is using apps or accounts, without your knowledge, in order to communicate.

7. Your child withdraws from the family and from friends.

The best preventative tool against this type of threat is to talk openly with your child. That means you need to move past your own discomfort and accept that they will probably feel uncomfortable too. This is not the time to sugar coat. Be truthful about the potential dangers, motives, and behaviors of sexual predators.

Instruct them to never give out their personal information online, and to never download pictures from anyone they don't know or have never met in person. Get them into the habit of questioning the motives of people who persistently seek them out or make suggestive comments to them.

Be sure to visit the website resources I gave you in chapter 7 and use their educational guides to help you. Some of them have examples of the things predators will say and do to groom and coerce children. You can also empower your child by teaching them how to spot or report a predator or any unsolicited suspicious behavior.

Remind them that accepting friend requests or followers on social media that they don't know puts them at risk. While you're at it, discuss how suggestive photos or flirtatious comments may attract predators. I know you may still feel like it's wrong to monitor your child's activity online, but let me leave you with this thought. You may not know of any parent who has had to deal with the pain of their child being victimized, but I do. I have sat with them as they cried and felt the burden of guilt and regret of not having done more. I guarantee you they would rather have dealt with their child's temporary anger instead of a lifetime of regret. Protect them now and they will understand later.

Protecting Your Child's Emotional & Physical Well-Being

As I mentioned before, the most effective way for you to protect your child is to be aware. You can do that by making routine observations, much in the same way that you look for signs and indicators that your child is sick. These can be physical changes in your child's appearance, changes in the way they engage socially, and behavioral changes in the way they act. Typically, if something is going on, you'll notice changes in all three areas. In social work, we often refer to this as an assessment of the "biopsychosocial" aspects of a client's life. It means you look at the physical, psychological, and social factors of a person's life in order to determine what type of help they may need. This type of assessment skill can also help you to parent.

Let's look at some of the common signs and indicators you should be on the lookout for.

Signs of Bullying	Signs of Self-Harming Behaviors
• Appears unusually sad, despondent, tearful, irritable, or distant	• Changes in dress; wears clothing to cover up arms and legs despite warm weather
• Noticeable shifts in mood, appetite, activity, or engagement with family members	• Appears unusually sad, despondent, tearful, irritable, or distant
• Starts to isolate or withdrawal from family and friends	• Noticeable shifts in mood, appetite, activity, or engagement with family members
• Changes online accounts, passwords, deletes profiles, account, or apps	• Starts to isolate or withdrawal from family and friends
• Makes excuses for not attending school	• Spends a considerable amount of time locked in room; insist on bedroom door being locked
• Develops headaches, stomachaches, or stress-related conditions	• Can become territorial over space and belongings
• Develops fear or resistance to walking to school or taking the bus	• Quick to get defensive and accusatory
• Decline in grades and school performance	• Lacks empathy, remorse, reaction and/or seems to be numb and "unfeeling"
• Torn, damaged or missing clothing, books, or belongings; unexplained injuries	• Cutting behaviors with razors, knives, pins, paperclips, or any sharp object
• Ask for money, steals money, or claims to have lost digital devices	• Unexplained scratches or cuts on arms, wrist, legs, or abdomen

Indicators of Suicidal Thoughts	Indicators of Drug/Alcohol Use
• History of symptoms of depression or anxiety (especially if child has been previously diagnosed with a psychiatric disorder)	• Appears withdrawn, depressed, tired, careless, and unconcerned about grooming or their appearance
• Uses or abuses drugs and alcohol as a way to escape or numb their pain	• Has become increasingly hostile, uncooperative, confrontational
• Previous victimization (experienced abuse, rape, neglect)	• Relationship with family members has deteriorated; breaks house rules
• Lacks a support system (has no friends and parent/child relationship is strained); unstable home life	• Teen has changed friends, you don't know teen's new friends, teen doesn't talk much about their new friends
• Experienced or exposed to a family member/friend who committed suicide	
• Under severe stress or recently experience trauma (death, significant loss, unplanned pregnancy, struggling with sexual identity, recent diagnoses)	• Drop in grades, decline in motivation at school, attendance has become irregular; loss of interest in hobbies
	• Teen has a difficult time concentrating; changes in eating and sleeping patterns
• Engages in risky or delinquent behaviors; has runaway in the past	• Items around the household go missing, teen constantly asking for money
• Has expressed or communicated thoughts of suicide, curiosity about death and the afterlife	• Uses body sprays, deodorizers, candles, mouthwash, or gum to cover up odors
• Expresses or shows feelings of hopelessness or defeat.	• Presence of rolling papers, bongs, homemade pipes, cans or plastic bottles

These lists are not exhaustive. Also, please note that if your child presents with a few or more signs, it is not confirmation of a problem. Think of the signs more as indicators that there MAY be a problem. Your goal is to gather information and take note of changes so that you can address your concerns with your child and a qualified professional. Addressing these signs immediately can make all the difference. Don't waste time blaming yourself or worrying about how this will affect the future. The most important thing is to take action; the sooner you do, the sooner you can start to help and heal.

Strategies to Protect Your Tweens & Teens

- **Stay aware.** Remember the greatest threats to your child's safety often occur in your home. It's smart to educate your children about talking to strangers, but don't forget that predators and bullies can access your child through digital devices. Also, consider what type of behavior you are role-modeling at home. Things like parental drug use, intimate partner violence, and emotional abuse can increase your child's risk of being victimization by a non-family member.

- **Get in their business.** It is your responsibility as a parent to monitor and supervise your child's life online. While tweens and teens are usually tech savvy, they still struggle with the emotional challenges and consequences of socializing online. Use parental controls and monitoring apps to help you identify and address issues of privacy and inappropriate behavior.

- **Set rules and boundaries.** Kids needs boundaries. Think of it like those bumpers you put in the gutters when you're first teaching your kid to bowl. They perform better when they have limits and it helps them to mature and practice accountability. In order for rules to be effective, you must be consistent with your consequences.

- **Be on the lookout for signs of an emotional issue.** Do not dismiss signs away as normal teen behavior. Talk openly with your child about the changes in their physical appearance, behavior, or social engagement. Instead of questioning the behavior, try to find the underlying emotion (like hurt, fear, anxiety, loss, grief, loneliness) that is fueling the behavior.

- **Recognize when you need professional help.** Don't burden yourself with the notion that you should be able to help your child. When your child is going through something, you are going through it with them and you both need the support of a professional. Seek help before matters get out of control. Especially in the case of drug use and depression.

Strategies for Protecting Young Children

- Talk to your kids about harmful things and people. Then repeat these talks over, and over, and over. You should be having conversations on such topics as: private parts, abductions, finding help when lost, what is an emergency, hazards in the home, and strangers just to name a few (visit my website, NourishedMinds.com, to get a copy of my guide *How to Talk to Your Kids About Sex & Safety*)

- Role play emergencies and situations with a potential "bad guy" who suggests something like inappropriate touching. You can also pretend to be the child and let them be the "bad guy," and walk them through how they can handle a situation.

- Have "dress rehearsals" where you create a mock unsafe situation to see how your child would react. Dateline did an episode like this where they had parents watching as hidden cameras recorded their children's reaction to an ice cream truck driver inviting them inside the van. Imagine the horror when some of the parents saw their kids get inside the van. Dress rehearsals are a great way to assess your child's safety skills without any real risk. I also suggest doing this with your child about getting lost. You can step away where they can't see you but you can see them and watch how they respond. They may get a little scared but I call that healthy fear, which you can use to really cement the lesson in their mind. Reunite with them and show them where they should go to meet you or get help if they ever really get lost.

- Create a safety kit that contains important items you will need in case of an emergency or crisis situation. Include: a recent photo of your child, medical records, a copy of immunization records, a copy of their birth certificate, a list of allergies, a fingerprint identification card, and a sample of your child's hair for DNA. Chances are you will probably never need to use this, but it will give you peace of mind knowing that you are prepared.

- Know your parental rights. Being an informed parent is the best way to ensure that you can protect your child. You should know your parental rights when it comes to your child's health, education, and their physical

[146]

safety. When you know your rights, it becomes much easier for you to advocate for your child's needs and people are way more likely to listen rather than dismiss you as being "overprotective."

Resources

CONSUMER GUIDES

Consumer Product Safety Commission
This site provides information on product recalls, and reports hazardous products and child protection safety issues.
www.cpsc.gov/

Good Guide
Here you will find safe, healthy, and green product reviews based on scientific ratings. *www.goodguide.com/*

Center for Science in the Public Interest
This helpful guide will help you to learn which food additives are safe and which ones you
need to avoid.
www.cspinet.org/reports/chemcuisine.htm

INTERNET SAFETY

Cyber Tip Hotline
Here is website and hotline for reporting child pornography or suspected child sexual exploitation
www.cybertipline.com/

Department of Justice
Here is a database of registered sex offenders
www.nsopw.gov/?AspxAutoDetectCookieSupport=1

TEENS

Phoenix House
This is a comprehensive list of the signs of teen drug use
www.phoenixhouse.org/prevention/signs-and-symptoms-of-substance-abuse/

Parent Guide to Teen Drug Use
www.teens.drugabuse.gov/
American Academy of Child & Adolescent Psychiatry's Guide on Bullying
www.aacap.org/AACAP/Families_and_Youth/Facts_for_Families/FFF-
Guide/Bullying-080.aspx

Web Wise Kids
This site contains great tips on social networking, cell phone dangers,
emerging technology, and instant messaging safety
www.webwisekids.org/

Safe 4 All
Resource for therapy, mentoring programs, and parent education
www.safe4all.org

YOUR RIGHTS

Education
Know your rights as a parent and the rights entitled to your child
www.ed.gov/policy/gen/guid/fpco/ferpa/index.html

Child Welfare
Child Welfare Information Gateway
Learn about your state laws regarding parental rights and child welfare
www.childwelfare.gov
Nourished Minds' Resource Guide
Get a copy of my complete guide of over 100 resources
www.NourishedMinds.com/resources

SAFETY KIT
Polly Klaus free child ID kit –
www.Pollyklaasaction.org/site/Advocacy?cmd=display&page=UserAction&
id=291

CH. 9 – IT TAKES A VILLAGE…AND AN OCCASIONAL GLASS OF WINE

What I'm about to say is the dot on the exclamation point of what I hope has been a mind-opening conversation between friends. I've said it before but it warrants saying again: I don't have any business telling you how to raise your kids. No one does. Every day we are unknowingly giving our power and control away to companies, governments, and other people. This is especially true in the case of parents like yourself who carry the added responsibility of raising and protecting our future generations. There is no more important job on this earth. It doesn't make any sense to make the job more complicated or stressful than it needs to be.

My hope is that my support will lighten your load. In fact, when I make an investment in your family's success, I am indirectly adding value to my world as well. Your happy, healthy, and informed children will grow up to be the holistic doctors, environmentally-friendly scientists, and anti-drug therapists who will one-day care for us aging adults. For that reason, I feel like you should have access to every tool, resource, and bit of advice and support you need.

I really tried to target those issues that seem to cause parents the most stress and fear. I've found that the more we know about something, the greater

[149]

the likelihood that we'll make confident choices and experience less uncertainty. I've also seen how effective these strategies can be. This is the same information and tools that I have used to help families successfully overcome daily challenges, as well as those unforeseeable life events. It's helped parents to avert crises and manage what initially had seemed to be an unmanageable situation. I'm hoping the greatest impact this book has on your parenting, however, is to remind you to *trust yourself.* If this book has inspired you to start asking more questions of the products you use and the healthcare you receive, then I have done my job.

Oh, and let us not forget the unsolicited advice from people who try to make you feel bad to make themselves feel better. That includes:

- *People who use intimidation or pressure to get you to buy or use something.*
- *Judgmental parents or friends who give you a guilt trip or always look for an opportunity to criticize your parenting.*
- *Women who question your choice to be a working mom or a stay-at-home mom.*
- *Organizations that try to push their agendas and beliefs onto you.*

These people will suck the life out of you if you let them. They will try to create doubt in you to make themselves feel superior. Don't give them any of your energy. Know that they are always coming from a place of wanting to hide from their own issues and insecurities. Strive to create a supportive village of like-minded parents and friends who share your values and beliefs. Don't be afraid to be that parent who is selective about their kid's food; who wants to meet the parent of their kid's friends; who refuses to buy harmful products; who questions the safety of vaccines; who chooses to see a holistic doctor; who decides to homeschool; or chooses a natural childbirth. Just do you and don't spend an ounce of your time worrying what other people think.

I also want to encourage you to be okay with making mistakes. Every parent makes mistakes and the occasional wrong choice. Empowered parenting isn't the absence of mistakes but the decision to learn from them. Don't try to be perfect—it's exhausting. Trust me, I know. I'm a recovering perfectionist. If I didn't learn to embrace failure, I never would have started my own practice or written a book.

Sure you're a parent, but you're also human. If one day you need to take a break from being proactive, then that's what you do. Stay on the couch for the day, go to the movies alone, or pour yourself a glass of wine and binge watch your favorite show. You deserve a break and if you don't allow yourself a few self-serving moments, your job of parenting will consume you.

I know we've covered a lot of ground in this book and trying to take it all in at once may be overwhelming. I don't want you thinking that you need to put all these strategies and ideas into action today. While this book may be ending: your journey of being an *Empowered Parent* has just begun. Here's a spoiler alert: it never really ends. That's because *Empowered Parenting* is a state of mind. It is the practice of maintaining your confidence and power through the sharp curves, deep dips, and confusing crossroads that come with the territory of being a parent.

You'll find that some of this information will serve you immediately. Other bits of information may lay dormant in your mind until you need it. I've also tried to write and organize this book in a way that will make it easy for you to reference it whenever life comes calling. So keep it handy.

Also keep in mind that I now consider you a part of my *Empowered Insiders Family* and hope that you will continue to visit with me at my website, workshops, and on social media. I invite you to share your thoughts and concerns with me, even if it's just to vent. I especially hope that you share any ideas you may have about topics, guides, books, or videos that you think I should create for parents like yourself. While I'm constantly researching and testing out new strategies, my most valuable experience and education has come from working and listening to parents. You have the ability to shape your children and to shape the world in which they live. Never forget your purpose. Never forget your power.

RESOURCE LIST

As a busy parent, I know you've got limited time to search for the information that you need. That's why I created this section which lists all the resources that I've noted throughout the book so that you can access them easily and at your convenience. Not all information is good information, so I conducted my own research to find websites and experts that are credible, with good reputations. If you'd like a copy of my Ultimate Resource Guide with over 100 listings for health, nutrition, consumer safety, healthcare, mental health, and more, then visit *www.NourishedMinds.com/resources*.

HEALTH CARE

Med Watch Safety Alerts
Helps consumers to stay informed on current safety issues with drugs, medical devices, and medical procedures
www.fda.gov/safety/medwatch/default.htm

Medication Guides
Provides consumers with information on comprehensive list of medications
and the serious adverse side effects from these medications
www.fda.gov/Drugs/DrugSafety/ucm085729.htm

New Pediatric Labeling Information Database
Database of drugs that the FDA has approved for use with children; lists recent
changes to labeling as well as findings from recent studies.
www.accessdata.fda.gov/scripts/sda/sdNavigation.cfm?sd=labelingdatabase

Society for Developmental & Behavioral Pediatrics
Find a clinician in your community that specializes in developmental issues
www.sdbp.org/resources/find-a-clinician.cfm

American Board of Integrative Holistic Medicine
Find an integrative holistic physician in your community
www.abihm.org/search-doctors

American Association of Naturopathic Physicians
Find a naturopathic physician in your community
www.naturopathic.org/AF_MemberDirectory.asp?version=2

VACCINES

Institute for Vaccine Safety
Independent reviews of vaccines and vaccine safety
www.vaccinesafety.edu/Aboutus.htm

National Vaccine Advisory Committee (NVAC)
Lists the latest reports on adult and child immunizations
www.hhs.gov/nvpo/nvac/reports/index.html

Center for Disease Control (CDC)
Links to recent research addressing the safety of vaccines and the questionable
link to autism
www.cdc.gov/vaccinesafety/pdf/cdcstudiesonvaccinesandautism.pdf

National Vaccine Information Center (NVIC)
Information on vaccine safety, schedules, and advice on adverse reactions
www.nvic.org

HOSPITALS/LABS/MEDICATIONS

State Medical Board Information
Assists you in researching your physician's conduct, license status, and experience
www.fsmb.org
www.Docinfo.org

Research Hospitals
www.medicare.gov/hospitalcompare/About/What-Is-HOS.html
www.whynotthebest.org
www.hospitalsafetyscore.org

Lab Test Online
Provides assistance with interpreting your lab results
www.labtestonline.org

Medication Guides
Comprehensive list of medications and the serious adverse side effects from these medications
www.fda.gov/Drugs/DrugSafety/ucm085729.htm

National Institute of Health
Comprehensive list of mental health medications
www.nimh.nih.gov/health/topics/mental-health-medications/index.shtml

Choose Wisely
Tool to help patients identify procedures and treatments that may be unnecessary or high risk
www.choosingwisely.org/doctor-patient-lists/

TECHNOLOGY

Common Sense Parenting
Content reviews for apps, movies, and games. Guidance and answers to your technology questions
www.CommonSenseParenting.org

Net Family News
A blog to educate and support parents on issues of internet safety and youth-related technology
www.NetFamilyNews.org

Connect Safely
Resources and tips on internet safety, privacy, and security
www.ConnectSafely.org

Net Smartz
Guides and videos on internet safety for kids and parents
www.NetSmartz.org

My Mobile Watchdog
Records text messages sent and received from your child's phone that you can print and review
www.mymobilewatchdog.com

Mobile Spy
Undetectable software you can load onto your child's phone which silently uploads data to your Mobile Spy account
www.mobile-spy.com

iProtect for iPhones
Monitoring system that logs instant message conversations; you can set it up to run at specific times
www.iprotectservices.com

CONSUMER GUIDES

Consumer Product Safety Commission
Information on product recalls, reporting hazardous products, and child protection safety issues
www.cpsc.gov/

Good Guide
Safe, healthy, and green product reviews based on scientific ratings
www.goodguide.com/

Center for Science in the Public Interest
Guide to learn which food additives are safe and which ones you need to avoid
www.cspinet.org/reports/chemcuisine.htm

INTERNET SAFETY

Cyber Tip Line
Website and hotline for reporting child pornography or suspected child sexual exploitation
www.cybertipline.com/

Database of registered sex offenders
www.nsopw.gov/?AspxAutoDetectCookieSupport=1

TEENS

Phoenix House
Comprehensive list of signs of teen drug use
www.phoenixhouse.org/prevention/signs-and-symptoms-of-substance-abuse/

Parent Guide to Teen Drug Use
www.teens.drugabuse.gov/

American Academy of Child & Adolescent Psychiatry
Guide on Bullying
www.aacap.org/AACAP/Families_and_Youth/Facts_for_Families/FFF-Guide/Bullying-080.aspx

Web Wise Kids
Tips on social networking, cell phone dangers, emerging technology, and instant messaging safety
www.webwisekids.org/

Safe 4 All
Resource for therapy, mentoring programs, and parent education
www.safe4all.org

EDUCATION

U.S. Department of Education
Know your rights as a parent and the rights entitled to your child
www.ed.gov/policy/gen/guid/fpco/ferpa/index.html

SAFETY KIT

Polly Klaus Free Child ID Kit
www.secure.pollyklaasaction.org/site/Advocacy?cmd=display&page=UserAction&id=291

Understanding Your Child's Characteristics By Age	
Social Characterstics Age 5- 7	• Like organized games and are very concerned about following rules. • Can be very competitive. May cheat at games. • Are very imaginative and involved in fantasy playing. • Are self-assertive, aggressive, want to be first, less cooperative than at five, and boastful. • Learn best through active participation.
Emotional Characteristics Age 5-7	• Are alert to feelings of others, but are unaware of how their own actions affect others. • Are very sensitive to praise and recognition. Feelings are easily hurt. • Inconsistent in level of maturity evidenced; regress when tired, often less mature at home • than with outsiders.
Mental Characteristics Age 5 -7	• Are very eager to learn. • Like to talk. • Their idea of fairness becomes a big issue. • Have difficulty making decisions.

[159]

Understanding Your Child's Characteristics By Age	
Social Characterstics Age 8-10	• Can be very competitive. • Are choosy about their friends. • Being accepted by friends becomes quite important. • Team games become popular. • Worshipping heroes, TV stars, and sports figures is common.
Emotional Characteristics Age 8-10	• Are very sensitive to praise and recognition. • Feelings are hurt easily. • Friends are very important during this time • Struggles with internal conflict between adults'rules and friend's rules.
Mental Characteristics Age 8-10	• The idea of fairness becomes a core issue for them. • Are eager to answer questions and show their knowledge. • Are very curious, and are collectors of things. • May go from one interest to the next after short time. • Want more independence. • Still desire parental support and guidance.

Understanding Your Child's Characteristics By Age

Social Characterstics Age 11-13	• Important to be accepted by friends. • Tend to gather in cliques both in and outside of school. • Interest in the form of crushes on members of the opposite sex. • Feel pressure to conform. May talk, dress, behave like peers in order to belong. • Concerned about what others say and think of them. • Employs manipulation to get their way.
Emotional Characteristics Age 11-13	• Need for praise and recognition. Sensitive to getting feelings hurt. • Internal conflict between parent's rules and friend's rules. • Struggle with desire to be treated like adult and still enjoy aspects of being a child. • Crucial time for developing self confidence and self esteem. • Look at the world more objectively and critical.
Mental Characteristics Age 11-13	• Want things to be perfect which can result in frustration after failed attempts. • Able to maintain longer attention span.

Understanding Your Child's Characteristics By Age	
Social Characterstics Age 14-16	• Friends set the rules of behavior. • Strong need to conform. • Attempt to belong by copying peers. • Very concerned what peers think about them. • Think in extreme terms, especially with emotions. • Afraid of being ridiculed and of being unpopular. • Prone to identify with an admired adult. • Interest in the opposite sex.
Emotional Characteristics Age 14-16	• Need for praise and recognition. • Sensitive to criticism. • Wants to be treated like an adult but still has childish ways. • Masks feelings of low self-esteem and lack of self confidence. • Looks at the world more objectively and critical.
Mental Characteristics Age 14-16	• Better understands moral principles. • Begins to self identify rather than being extension of peers and parents.

BIBLIOGRAPHY

CHAPTER 1

American Humane Association. 2005. *AmericanHumane.org.* Accessed March 4, 2015. http://www.americanhumane.org/children/stop-child-abuse/fact-sheets/child-abuse-and-neglect-statistics.html.

CHAPTER 2

Ariely, Dan. 2008. *Predictably Irrational: The Hidden Forces That Shape Our Decisions.* New York: Harper.

Barquet, Nicolau. 1997. "Smallpox: The Triumph over the Most Terrible of the Ministers of Death." *Annals of Internal Medicine* 635.

Federal Interagency Forum. 2015. *America's Children: Key Indicators of Well-Being.* Washington, D.C.: Government Printing Office.

Hanson, A. 2013. "The Future of Convenience Stores: Food Destination." *Convenience Store News,* May 19.

Hunter, Diane. 2009. *Food Smart: Understanding Nutrition in the 21st Century.* Consumer Press.

Mahon, Mary. 2014. *Commonwealthfund.org.* June 16. Accessed May 4, 2016. http://www.commonwealthfund.org/publications/press-releases/2014/jun/us-health-system-ranks-last.

Multisponsor Surveys, Inc. 2012. *www.multisponsor.com.* Accessed July 14, 2-14. http://www.multisponsor.com/index.php/category/research-update/food-and-beverage.

O'Reilly, Andrea. 2013. "Why the 1970s Were the Best Time to Be a Mom." *The Globe and Mail,* April 15.

[163]

Safekids Worldwide. 2015. "Medicine Safety for Children: An In-Depth Look at Calls to Poison Centers." *www.safekids.org*. March. Accessed February 13, 2016. http://www.safekids.org/research-report/medicine-safety-children-depth-look-calls-poison-centers-march-2015.

Sifferlin, Alexandra. 2015. "Americans Spent a Record Amount on Medicine in 2014." *Time*, April 14.

Sloan, E. 2014. "What, WHere, and When America Eats." *Food Technology*, January.

Statista. 2010. *Statista.com*. Accessed February 10, 2016. http://www.statista.com/topics/1660/food-retail/.

—. 2013. *Statista.com*. Accessed February 10, 2016. http://www.statista.com/topics/1496/snack-foods/.

—. 2012. *Statista.com*. Accessed February 10, 2016.

—. 2012. *Statista.com*. Accessed February 10, 2016. https://www.statista.com/chart/3967/which-countries-pay-the-most-for-medicinal-drugs/.

Technomic. 2013. *Technomic.com*. Accessed December 11, 2016. https://www.technomic.com/Reports_and_Newsletters/Industry_Reports/dyn_PubLoad_v2.php?pID=1.

U.S. Census Bureau. 2010. *America's Families and Living Arrangements*. Accessed July 6, 2014. https://www.census.gov/population/www/socdemo/hh-fam/cps2010.html.

For more information about the topics presented in Chapter 2:

Bird, Adrian. "Perceptions of Epigenetics." *Nature* 447, no. 7143 (2007): 396-98.doi:10.1038/nature05913.

Substance Abuse and Mental Health Services Administration, Drug Abuse
Warning Network, 2011: *National Estimates of Drug-Related
Emergency Department Visits*. HHS Publication No. (SMA) 13-
4760, DAWN Series D-39. Rockville, MD: Substance Abuse and
Mental Health Services Administration, 201.

Full Report and Key Findings: The 2012 Partnership Attitude Tracking
Study, Sponsored by MetLife Foundation - Partnership for Drug-Free
Kids." *Partnership for Drug-Free Kids*. April 23, 2013. Accessed
November 13, 2015. http://www.drugfree.org/newsroom/full-report-
and-key-findings-the-2012-partnership-attitude-tracking-study-
sponsored-by-metlife-foundation/.

U.S. Health in International Perspective: Shorter Lives, Poorer Health." *The
National Academies Press*. Accessed February 13, 2016.
http://www.nap.edu/catalog.php?record_id=13497.

CHAPTER 3

Centers for Disease Control and Prevention. 2013. "CDC.gov." *Trends in
Foodborne Illness in the United States, 2012*. Accessed February 13,
2015. http://www.cdc.gov/Features/dsFoodNet2012/index.html.

Druker, Steven. 2004. "Why Concerns About Health Risks of Genetically
Engineered Food Are Scientifically Justified." *Allience for Bio-
Integrity*. Alliance for Bio-Integrity.Environmental Working Group.
2015. *www.ewg.org*. Accessed October 19, 2015.
http://www.ewg.org/foodnews/faq.php.

Food and Agricultural Organization. 2015. *Status of World's Soil Resources*.
Food and Agricultural Organization of the United Nations.
http://www.fao.org/documents/card/en/c/c6814873-efc3-41db-b7d3-
2081a10ede50/.

Forman, Joel, and Janet Silverstein. 2012. "Organic Foods: Health and Environmental Advantages and Disadvantages." *Pediatrics* 1406-1415.

Hunter, Diane. 2009. *Food Smart: Understanding Nutrition in the 21st Century.* Consumer Press.

Institute for Responsible Technology. 2014. *GMO Myths and Truths.* Institute for Responsible Technology. http://gmomythsandtruths.earthopensource.org.

Marler, J., and J. Wallin. 2006. *Human Health, the Nutritional Quaity of Harvested Food.* Whitepaper, Nutrition Security Institute. Accessed December 3, 2015. http://www.nutritionsecurity.org/PDF/NSI_White Paper_Web.pdf.

Poti, J.M., Michelle A Mendez, Shu Wen Ng, and Barry M Popkin. 2015. "Is the degree of food processing and convenience linked with the nutritional quality of foods purchased by US households?" *Journal of Clinical Nutrition* 1251-1262.

Robbins, John. 2001. *The Food Revolution: How Your Diet Can Help Save Your Life and the World.* Berkeley: Conari Press.

The Economist. 2014. "Milking Taxpayers: As Crop Prices Fall, Farmers Grow Subsidies Instead." *The Economist*, October 19. http://www.economist.com/news/united-states/21643191-crop-prices-fall-farmers-grow-subsidies-instead-milking-taxpayers.

For more information about the topics presented in Chapter 3:

Andrews, David. Natural vs. Artificial Flavors. *Environmental Working Group.* Accessed December 11, 2015. http://www.ewg.org/foodscores/content/natural-vs-artificial-flavors.

[166]

Balch, J., M.D. and P. Balch, CNC. *Prescription for Nutritional Healing* (4th Ed). New York, NY: Penguin Group. 2006.

Holford, Patrick. *The New Optimum Nutrition Bible*. Berkeley, CA: Crossing Press. 2004.

Squires, D., and C. Anderson. "U.S. Health Care from a Global Perspective: Spending, Use of Services, Prices, and Health in 13 Countries." The Commonwealth Fund, October 2015.

Zand, J., R. Walton, and B. Rountree, *Smart Medicine for a Healthier Child: A practical A-to-Z reference to natural and conventional treatments for infants and children*. Garden City Park, New York: Avery Publishing Group.1994.

CHAPTER 4

Deyo, PhD, Richard A., and Donald Patrick, PhD. 2006. *Hope or Hype: The Obsession with Medical Advances and the High Cost of False Promises*. New York: American Management Association.

Mackey, T.K., and B.A. Liang. 2015. "It's Time to Shine the Light on Direct-to-Consumer Advertising." *The Annals of Family Medicine* 82-85.

Shannon, Scott M. 2012. *Parenting the Whole Child; a holistic child psychiatrist offers practical wisdom on behavior, brain health, nutrition, exercise, family life, peer relationships, school life, trauma, medications, and more*. New York: Norton & Company.

For more information about the topics presented in Chapter 4:

American Psychological Association. "Psychopharmological, Psychosocial, and Combined Interventions for Childhood Disorders: Evidence base, contextual factors, and future directions." *American Psychological Association Working Group on Psychoactive*

[167]

Medications for Children and Adolescents. Washington, DC: American Psychological Association. 2006.

Fitzgerald, Randall. *The Hundred Year Lie: How food and medicine are destroying your health.* New York: Penguin Group. 2006.

Healy, David. *Pharmageddon.* Berkeley, CA: University of California Press. 2012.

Waxman HA. The lessons of Vioxx—drug safety and sales. *New England Journal of Medicine.* 2005;352(25):2576–2578. [PubMed].

ProCon.org. "35 FDA-Approved Prescription Drugs Later Pulled from the Market - Prescription Drug Ads – ProCon.org." *ProConorg Headlines.* Accessed March 02, 2016. http://prescriptiondrugs.procon.org/view.resource.php?resourceID=0 05528.

Kalikow, Kevin. *Your Child in the Balance: An Insider's Guide for Parents to the Psychiatric Medicine Dilemma.* MA: 2006.

CHAPTER 5

Baxby, Derek. 2001. *Smallpox Vaccine: Ahead of Its Time.* Berkeley, U.K.: Jenner Museum.

Colgrove, James. 2006. *State of immunity: The politics of vaccination in twentieth century America.* Berkeley: University of California Press.

Fenn, Elizabeth. 2001. *Pox Americana: The Great Smallpox Epidemic of 1775-82.* New York: Hill and Wang.

O'Shea, T. *The Sanctity of Human Blood: Vaccination is not Immunization.* Denver, Colorado: New West. 2009.

For more information about the topics presented in Chapter 5:

Tenpenny. *Vaccine Titer Test.* Accessed May 16, 2016.
http://drtenpenny.com/titer-test-information/titer-tests/.

Vax Truth. "History of Infectious Disease and Vaccination in the United States." *Vax Truth.* August 29, 2011. Accessed February 16, 2016. http://vaxtruth.org/2011/08/history-of-infectious-disease-and-vaccination-in-the-united-states/.

CHAPTER 6

Administration, Substance Abuse and Mental Health Services. 2012. "Mental Health, United States, 2010." *Substance Abuse and Mental Health Services Administration.* Rockville: US HHS.

American Diabetes Association. 2014. *Diabetes.org.* Accessed March 2, 2016. http://www.diabetes.org/diabetes-basics/statistics/.

Centers for Disease Control. 2016. *CDC.gov.* Accessed March 2, 2016. http://www.diabetes.org/diabetes-basics/statistics/.

Federal Interagency Forum. 2015. *America's Children: Key Indicators of Well-Being.* Washington, D.C.: Government Printing Office.

Fitzgerald, Randall. *The Hundred Year Lie: How food and medicine are destroying your health.* New York: Penguin Group. 2006

Mahon, Mary. 2014. *Commonwealthfund.org.* June 16. Accessed May 4, 2016. http://www.commonwealthfund.org/publications/press-releases/2014/jun/us-health-system-ranks-last.

Ng, Marie. 2013. "Global, regional, and national prevalence of overweight and obesity in children and adults during 1980–2013: a systematic analysis for the Global Burden of Disease Study 2013." *The Lancet* 766-781.

Ogden, MD, CL, B.K. Kit, and K.M. Flegal. 2014. "Prevalence of Childhood and Adult Obesity in the United States." *Journal of the American Medical Association* 806-814.

For more information about the topics presented in Chapter 6:

Choosing Wisely. "Doctor, Patient Lists." Accessed March 23, 2016. http://www.choosingwisely.org/doctor-patient-lists/.

Fitzgerald, Randall. *The Hundred Year Lie: How food and medicine are destroying your health.* New York: Penguin Group. 2006

Hendel, Amy. *Fat Families, Thin Families: How to Save Your Family from the Obesity Trap.* Dallas, Texas: BenBella Books. 2008.

Johnston, L. D., O'Malley, P. M., Bachman, J. G., & Schulenberg, J. E. (2013). Monitoring the Future national results on drug use: 2012 Overview, Key Findings on Adolescent Drug Use. Ann Arbor: *Institute for Social Research*, The University of Michigan.

Malone, Patrick. *The Life You Save: Nine Steps to Finding the Best Medical Care—And Avoiding the Worst.* Cambridge, MA: Da Capo Press. 2009.

Substance Abuse and Mental Health Services Administration. (2012). *Mental Health, United States, 2010.* HHS Publication No. (SMA) 12-4681. Rockville, MD: Substance Abuse and Mental Health Services Administration.

CHAPTER 7

The National Campaign to Prevent Teen and Unplanned Pregnancy. 2014. "Teen Sexting Study." *The National Campaign to Prevent Teen and Unplanned Pregnancy.* October.

For more information about the topics presented in Chapter 7:

Anderson, Monica. "Parents, Teens and Digital Monitoring." *Pew Research Center Internet Science Tech* RSS. 2016. Accessed March 30, 2016. http://www.pewinternet.org/2016/01/07/parents-teens-and-digital monitoring/.

Legal Shield. "Protect Your Kids from Cyberbullies." *Legal News*. Accessed September 20, 2015. http://connect.legalshield.com/hubfs/member_newsletter/August_20 15/PVIssue10_v4.pdf.

Rainie, Lee. "13 Things to Know About Teens and Technology." *Pew Research Center Internet Science Tech* RSS. 2014. Accessed March 30, 2016.

http://www.pewinternet.org/2014/07/23/13-things-to-know-about-teens-and-technology/.

The Federal Trade Commission. *Heads Up: Stop, Think, Connect*. July 2013. OnGuard Online.Gov.

The Federal Trade Commission. *Net Cetera: Chatting with Kids About Being Online*. January 2014. OnGuard Online.Gov.

CHAPTER 8

Flores, J. Robert. 2002. "National Incidence Studies of Missing, Abducted, Runaway, and Thrownaway Children in America." *NISMART Bulletin*. Office of Juvenile, October.

For more information about the topics presented in Chapter 8:

Finkelhor, D., H. Hammer, and A. Seldak. "NISMART Bulletin: Runaway/Thrownaway Children: National Estimates and Characteristics." *U.S. Department of Justice, Office of Justice Programs, Office of Juvenile Justice and Delinquency Prevention.*

2002. Accessed May 04, 2016.
https://www.ncjrs.gov/html/ojjdp/nismart/04.

Centers for Disease Control and Prevention. "Children, the Flu, and the Flu
Vaccine." *Centers for Disease Control and Prevention.* August 21,
2015. Accessed February 03, 2016.

Christian, C. W., and R. D. Sege. "Child Fatality Review." *Pediatrics* 126,
no. 3 (2010): 592-96. Accessed April 11, 2016.
doi:10.1542/peds.2010-2006.
http://www.cdc.gov/flu/protect/children.htm.

National Institute on Alcohol Abuse and Alcoholism. "Underage Drinking."
National Institute on Alcohol Abuse and Alcoholism (NIAAA).
Accessed April 2, 2016. http://niaaa.nih.gov/alcohol-health/special-
populations-co-occurring-disorders/underage-drinking.

Seals, N. "Compulsive Sexual Behavior: Paraphilic Type --
Pedophilia." Social Work Reference Guide (November 13,
2015): *Social Work Reference Center*, EBSCO*host.* Retrieved
January 12, 2016.

www.ingramcontent.com/pod-product-compliance
Lightning Source LLC
LaVergne TN
LVHW021448080426
835509LV00018B/2209